CWLA Best Practice Guidelines

D1270801

CHILD WELFARE LEAGUE OF AMERICA

WASHINGTON, DC

This publication was made possible by a grant from the Administration for Children, Youth and Families, Children's Bureau, Washington, DC (Federal Grant #90-XA-0061).
An Executive Summary for this document is available online at www.cwla.org.

The Child Welfare League of America is the nation's oldest and largest membership-based child welfare organization. We are committed to engaging people everywhere in promoting the well-being of children, youth, and their families, and protecting every child from harm.

CHILD WELFARE LEAGUE OF AMERICA, INC.
HEADQUARTERS
440 First Street, NW, Third Floor, Washington, DC 20001-2085
E-mail: books@cwla.org

CURRENT PRINTING (last digit)
10 9 8 7 6 5 4 3 2 1

Cover and text design by Jennifer R. Geanakos
Edited by Julie Gwin and Eve Malakoff-Klein

Printed in the United States of America

ISBN-10: 1–58760-071-4
ISBN-13: 978-1-58760-071-5

Library of Congress Cataloging-in-Publication Data
CWLA best practice guidelines : children missing from care / Child Welfare League of America.
　　p. cm.
　Includes bibliographical references.
　ISBN-13: 978-1-58760-071-5 (pbk. : alk. paper)
　ISBN-10: 1-58760-071-4 (pbk. : alk. paper)
　1. Runaway children--United States. 2. Missing children--United States. 3. Kidnapping--United States--Prevention. 4. Social work with children--United States. 5. Social work with youth--United States. I. Child Welfare League of America.
　HV741.C858 2005
　362.7--dc22
　　　　　　　　　　2005011684

Contents

Dedication

These best practice guidelines are dedicated to Rilya Shenise Wilson, a young girl who was last seen by her caregiver in January 2001 at age 4 while in the care and custody of the Florida Department of Children and Families. The publicity following Rilya's disappearance unearthed an erosion in child safety across our nation's public child welfare system—children missing from care.

As of this writing, Rilya has not been located...she is a painful and poignant reminder that we are entrusted to protect children from harm when their families or caregivers are unable or unwilling to do so. We hope the guidance that follows will lead the way for the provision of quality, systematic, coordinated practices by child welfare and law enforcement professionals so that we can, whenever possible, prevent the initial occurrence of missing children and so that we can effectively respond to, recover, and safely return all children once they go missing from our care.

The story of Rilya Wilson's life is a clarion call for us all. We must not let children who go missing be forgotten. For Rilya—and for all the children and youth in our care—we are the watchdogs of their safety and the trustees of their future opportunities and promise. Rilya, we will forever remember.

Introduction

The Child Welfare League of America (CWLA), in collaboration with the National Center for Missing & Exploited Children® (NCMEC), has developed best practice guidelines to provide agencies with an effective tool to develop administrative policies, procedures, and case practices that will decrease the likelihood of children going missing from out-of-home care; assure a coordinated and effective response to instances in which children do go missing; and ensure that once children are returned to care, they, their caregivers, and their birthfamilies receive the necessary and appropriate services and supports for recovery and resolution.

CWLA is a national membership organization of nearly 900 child-serving agencies throughout North America. Its public and voluntary agency members serve children, youth, and families in need of child protective services, family preservation and support services, kinship care, foster care, independent living, residential group care, adoption, pregnancy services, parenting skills, mental health treatment, substance abuse treatment, child day care, housing, and juvenile justice services, as well as other essential supports and services. CWLA's mission is to engage people everywhere in promoting the well-being of children, youth, and families and protecting every child from harm.

Congress mandated NCMEC in 1984 to provide services nationwide for families and professionals in preventing the abduction, endangerment, and sexual exploitation of children. The center:

- serves as a clearinghouse of information about missing and exploited children;

- operates a CyberTipline that the public may use to report Internet-related child sexual exploitation;

- provides technical assistance to individuals and law enforcement agencies in the prevention, investigation, prosecution, and treatment of cases involving missing and exploited children;

- assists the U.S. Department of State in certain cases of international child abduction in accordance with the Hague Convention on the Civil Aspects of International Child Abduction;

- offers training programs to law enforcement and social service professionals;

- distributes photographs and descriptions of missing children worldwide;

- coordinates child-protection efforts with the private sector;

- networks with nonprofit service providers and state clearinghouses about missing-persons cases; and

- provides information about effective state legislation to help ensure the protection of children.

Importance of This Issue

These best practice guidelines grew out of the need to go beyond current resources and respond to new developments in the field. High-profile cases have heightened awareness and visibility of the consequences when agencies do not prevent missing-from-care episodes. Several states have experienced damaging publicity in the wake of cases in which children have gone missing from care. In Florida, the failure to locate 5-year-old Rilya Wilson in 2002 brought national attention to a state child welfare system that was unable to determine the location of almost 400 children. As a result, several states began efforts to make sure they could account for the whereabouts of all their children in care—and it became apparent that Florida was not alone in its inability to locate large numbers of children. Both before and after the disclosure of Rilya's disappearance, several states dealt with cases in which young people who ran away from care were found murdered, victims of the dangers faced by runaways living on the street. The attention given to such cases has served to focus national attention on both runaways and child welfare systems unable to keep track of the children in their care.

The child welfare field needs consistent, quality practices to prevent, respond to, and resolve missing-from-care episodes. No uniform guidelines exist for these processes, and practices vary across state agencies. This volume provides agencies and workers with guidelines to help reduce the number of episodes, minimize the distress experienced by birthfamilies and caregivers during the episodes, and achieve better resolutions for all parties once children are located.

Child welfare agencies need clear lines of communication and coordinated practices to guide their interaction with law enforcement agencies that are concurrently involved in missing episodes. Concurrent with the publication of these guidelines, NCMEC is providing law enforcement agencies with companion guidelines and tools to aid in the investigation, recovery, and reunification of children missing from out-of-home care. CWLA's best practice guidelines give child welfare agencies and workers direction in partnerships that adhere to good social work practice while enabling law enforcement agencies to investigate and resolve cases in accordance with their own procedures.

Project Overview

For FY 2004, CWLA was the recipient of a one-year grant, pursuant to the legislative authority of the Child Abuse Prevention and Treatment Act (CAPTA), to improve the safety and well-being of children in out-of-home care. In collaboration with NCMEC, CWLA was to provide comprehensive guidance to child welfare and law enforcement agencies on monitoring the status of children in the custody of the child welfare agency and responding when any of the children are missing. CWLA and NCMEC developed and are disseminating these coordinated guidelines to enhance the capacity to monitor the whereabouts and safety of children in foster care and to effectively respond when a child in care is missing.

The Children Missing from Care Project is a response to the heightened awareness of the risk of harm faced by children who go missing from the agency's care, whether due to their overt actions (i.e., running away), the actions of others (i.e., being abducted), or the inattentiveness of the custodial agency (i.e., being "lost" in care). A coordinated response by child welfare and law enforcement is the best hope for reducing these risks. The initiative was developed to accomplish this goal through four objectives:

1. Clarify the definitions of terms related to "children missing from care" and identify data elements that agencies should collect and aggregate.

2. Explore the scope of the problem, identifying patterns and trends and delineating the individual, institutional, and environmental factors that affect the problem.

3. Develop practice guidelines for child welfare and law enforcement professionals.

4. Disseminate guidance to child welfare and law enforcement agencies through articles, conference presentations, and the NCMEC and CWLA websites.

The Need for Best Practice Guidelines

Child safety has long been a primary focus of child welfare. With the passage of the Adoption and Safe Families Act of 1997 (ASFA), the federal government underscored the importance of safety, permanence, and well-being in the delivery of all child welfare services, including foster care. When a child enters out-of-home care and at some point goes missing, all three of these essential outcomes are jeopardized:

- Child safety is the first and most immediate concern. Whether the child has been abducted by a nonfamily member, has been taken by a family member (frequently back into the environment previously deemed unsafe), or runs away, the child's very life is potentially in danger. Even if no immediate danger exists, the risks of leaving care, particularly for runaways, include violence, sexual victimization or exploitation, substance abuse, and criminal offending. (Biehal & Wade, 1999)

- Permanence may be compromised when foster families rethink their commitment to young people who run from their care, and it may become difficult to find a permanent family for children who have a history of running. Children who run away or are abducted, even by a family member, may lose connections with parents, siblings, extended family, or other significant adults.

- The well-being of children in out-of-home care is measured by the federal government in terms of the ability of all families to provide for the needs of their children as well as in terms of the appropriateness and adequacy of the educational and health services the children receive (U.S. Department of Health and Human Services [DHHS], 2000); by these measures, agencies cannot even assess the well-being of any missing child. It is safe to say, however, that the emotional, educational, health, and other needs of missing children are rarely met during the missing episode and that such breaks in care often have long-term negative effects. The Runaway and Homeless Youth Act of 1974 (RHYA), as Amended by the Missing, Exploited, and Runaway Children Protection Act (P.L. 106-71), recognized that runaways "are at risk of developing serious health and other problems because they lack sufficient resources to obtain care and may live on the street for extended periods thereby endangering themselves" (Section 302[1], p. 1) and "have a disproportionate share of health, behavioral, and emotional problems compared to the general population of youth, but have less access to health care and other appropriate services." (Section 302[6], p. 2)

Child welfare agencies have a duty to ensure the safety, permanence, and well-being of the children for whom they are responsible. Clearly, they cannot do so when children are missing for any reason. Agencies have a responsibility to prevent missing-from-care episodes, respond quickly and in partnership with law enforcement agencies when children do go missing, and provide the resources and services necessary to bring each case to a successful resolution once they locate the child.

Some states and agencies do maintain accurate records and have well-developed policies and practices for the prevention of, response to, and resolution of missing episodes. Others do not, however, and practices are often inconsistent in and across jurisdictions. The field needs more guidance to inform these processes at the state, county, and local levels. CWLA's best practice guidelines are intended to provide such guidance.

The Relationship Between CWLA Standards of Excellence and Best Practice Guidelines

CWLA's *Standards of Excellence* are goals for the continuing improvement of services for children and their families. As goal standards, they reflect what the field collectively recognizes as the best ways to meet children's and families' needs. They provide a vision to which agencies and workers can aspire.

CWLA's *Best Practice Guidelines* elaborate on and operationalize practice standards by providing more specific, detailed guidance for agencies and practitioners. As with practice standards, guidelines are informed by experts and represent the best thinking of professionals across relevant program areas.

They are not intended to provide step-by-step instructions on, for example, how to respond when a youth runs away from care. Rather, these guidelines identify specific issues that require consideration and activities that child placement agencies should undertake when a child is missing from placement.

The Guidelines Development Process

Before beginning to develop these guidelines, CWLA undertook three preliminary activities—the development of an issue brief, administration of a survey of the National Working Group to Improve Child Welfare Data, and convening an expert panel.

Issue Brief

CWLA staff conducted a literature search, interviewed key informants, and identified promising practices to describe and analyze the current state of knowledge regarding children missing from care, including the causative factors and prospective remedies. The resulting issue brief is intended to inform federal, state, and local policy makers as well as members of the law enforcement and child welfare communities of that which is both known and unknown about children missing from care and to provide formative guidance in the development of these guidelines (Kaplan, 2004). It includes a discussion of definitional issues and recommended practice and policy strategies relevant to the prevention of episodes and response to, recovery of, and return of children missing from care.

Survey

In November 2003, CWLA contacted members of the National Working Group to Improve Child Welfare Data, a state-driven entity established to identify common definitions, patterns, and differences in state child welfare data; better understand the data and how they reflect practice; and ultimately achieve standardization in selected areas. CWLA asked the group to respond to a survey about state child welfare agency definitions, policies, and practices regarding missing and runaway children. Specific topics included:

- state definitions of *missing* and *runaway* as these terms apply to children and youth in out-of-home care,

- the use of agency management information systems to track and monitor children who are missing from care, and

- coordination between child welfare management information systems and the federal National Crime Information Center (NCIC).

CWLA received responses from 24 states. The information proved invaluable in identifying strong practices, particularly in the areas of tracking and monitoring missing children through the use of automated data systems. The survey responses also pointed out state-to-state inconsistencies and areas in need of practice development. These guidelines seek to address those areas.

Expert Panel Meeting

In March 2004, CWLA convened a meeting to hear from national experts in child welfare, law enforcement, research and data, policy, and the judiciary with specialized expertise in issues related to children missing from care. Participants included individuals with a range of knowledge, skills, and perspectives. The discussion informed and enriched these guidelines.

The Scope of These Best Practice Guidelines

The field has a dearth of research about children who go missing from out-of-home care. Little examination has been devoted to the identification of best practices—or even promising practices—in the prevention of, response to, and resolution of missing-from-care episodes. Therefore, these best practice guidelines are informed primarily by information identified in CWLA's *Children Missing from Care* issue brief (Kaplan, 2004), guidance provided by participants at the expert meeting CWLA held in March 2004, and CWLA's *Standards of Excellence* in the areas of services for abused and neglected children and their families (1999b), family foster care services (1995), kinship care services (1999a), residential services (2004b), and transition, independent living, and self-sufficiency services (2005). The guidelines specifically note cases in which research provides evidence-based guidance for practice.

These best practice guidelines provide direction to child placement agencies responsible for children in out-of-home care, both in family foster care and in group and residential settings. They were prepared in conjunction and go hand in hand with guidelines for law enforcement agencies on children missing from care.

Chapter 1 lays the groundwork for the practice guidelines that follow by:

- establishing a set of definitions regarding children missing from care, including children who run, children who are abducted, and children who are "lost" in care, to enable child welfare and law enforcement agencies to communicate more efficiently and effectively; and

- describing those aspects of what is known about the unique characteristics of each of these categories of children that affects child welfare practice and law enforcement response.

Chapter 2 addresses the quality management and administration issues facing child welfare agencies, including:

- the legal context for the guidelines;

- key policy and practice issues, including systemic concerns related to each of the categories of children missing from care, training, and the recruitment and retention of foster parents;

- child welfare agency record-keeping practices that both reduce the incidence of children being lost in care and contribute to the speedier recovery of children who do go missing;

- interjurisdictional matters;

- balancing the need for maintaining the confidentiality of children in out-of-home care and their families with the need to share information with law enforcement agencies and the media;

- coordination of efforts with other community partners whose involvement can contribute to the safety of all children, including those in out-of-home care; and

- comprehensive agency planning as a tool that affects all phases of missing-from-care episodes, from prevention through return and resolution.

Chapter 3 discusses partnership issues between child welfare and law enforcement agencies that affect the recovery and return of children missing from care, including:

- the legal context for law enforcement policy and practice,

- responsibilities of law enforcement agencies in missing-children cases,

- the resources and services law enforcement agencies provide,

- key elements in the partnership between child welfare and law enforcement agencies,

- coordination between information systems employed by law enforcement to track the status of missing children and by child welfare agencies to maintain data on all children in their care, and

- the development of memoranda of understanding to provide clear and specific delineation of responsibilities in dealing with missing children cases.

Chapter 4 addresses the prevention of missing from care episodes by focusing on elements of good child welfare practice that serve to maintain children and youth safely in the care of the agency. It includes discussion of:

- the agencies and individuals who contribute to and are responsible for the safety of children and youth in care and the prevention of missing episodes;

- the role of proper preparation of children, their caregivers, and their families in the prevention of episodes;

- the safety and risk assessments that identify and address potential concerns;

- the contribution of placement selection and placement stability to maintaining children safely in out-of-home care;

- practices that support placement stability and the prevention of missing-from-care episodes; and

- the role of information technology in the prevention of missing-from-care episodes.

Chapter 5 covers the responses to cases in which children are missing from care, including:

- recommendations for handling all missing-from-care cases through single points of contact in both child welfare and law enforcement agencies;

- necessary notifications when a child has gone missing;

- assessment of the risk factors that may affect the child's safety during the episode;

- the investigation;

- interjurisdictional issues;

- the potential involvement of juvenile justice agencies;

- the role of information technology in the response to and investigation of missing-from-care episodes; and

- provision of ongoing support to the child's caregiver, birthfamily, and other children in care while the child is missing.

Chapter 6 addresses the practices and activities that should occur after the child is located, including:

- roles and responsibilities of the child welfare and law enforcement agencies in the return of the child to the physical custody of the child welfare agency;

- individuals and agencies to be notified about the child's recovery;

- return of the child to the same or another foster family or placement; and

- issues to be dealt with in a debriefing interview with the child.

CHAPTER 1

Children Who Go Missing: An Overview

It is essential to establish a shared understanding of issues and a common language relevant to children who go missing from out-of-home care both within the ranks of the child welfare agency and with law enforcement professionals and their host agencies. This includes a common language to define missing episodes in a consistent manner, an understanding of some of the common reasons children run away from out-of-home care, the risks associated with running, and the issues involved in cases of abduction by a family member when children are in the care of the state.

This chapter's definitions are intended to facilitate a common language and partnership for all agencies involved with missing children, particularly those child welfare and law enforcement professionals who are involved in the prevention, recovery, and resolution of instances of children missing from care. The fact that a given child's situation falls into one of the definitional categories does not automatically prescribe a course of action for either the child welfare agency or the law enforcement agency. The definitions used are informed by the work of participants at an expert panel meeting (CWLA, 2004a) and by existing U.S. Department of Justice National Incidence Studies of Missing, Abducted, Runaway and Thrownaway Children–2 (NISMART-2) definitions (Sedlak, Finkelhor, Hammer, & Schultz, 2002). These guidelines provide compatible definitions developed by NCMEC for use by law enforcement personnel in the response to missing-from-care episodes. In addition, definitions used by individual law enforcement and child welfare agencies can and should depend on the statutes in the states where those agencies are located.

A child is considered *missing from care* if he or she is not in the physical custody of the child welfare agency or the person or institution with whom the agency placed the child. The whereabouts of the missing child may be known or unknown. This umbrella category includes children who have run away, are abducted from care, or are lost in care.

Children Who Run

A child is considered a runaway if he or she is voluntarily missing for 12 hours or overnight.* This definition does *not* preclude the possibility that a child may be considered a runaway *sooner than 12 hours or overnight*. Foster parents, custodians, and other caregivers must report a child as missing as soon as they have reason to believe that a child has run from care. Under no circumstances should any caregivers forestall the reporting of a child who may have run away beyond 12 hours or overnight. Circumstances and child characteristics under which a child may be considered a runaway sooner than by the above definition include:

- The child has declared that he or she is running away, either directly to the caregiver or through another party, such as a friend or other child in the placement.

- The child misses a clearly stated deadline or curfew and the caregiver has reason to believe the child does not intend to return.

- The child or another party contacts the caregiver or social worker, saying that he or she is not returning.

- Some or all of the child's possessions, such as clothing, are missing.

- The child is of school age or younger, physically or developmentally disabled, or emotionally or mentally impaired.

- The child has recently been placed in care.

- The child has a history of runaway behavior.

Reasons for Running

Children and youth run away from out-of-home care for many reasons, but most runaways fall into a few categories:

- According to NISMART, when children run, it is often to escape protracted and painful family conflict, or physical, sexual, or psychological abuse. (Hammer, Finkelhor, & Sedlak, 2002)

- Some youth are lured away by adults who will exploit them once they are outside the control and care of their placement. These children are at great risk of being victimized physically and sexually.

---

* The National Center on Missing & Exploited Children advises all parents and caregivers to immediately report children who are missing to law enforcement.

- Some children leave care to be with some other person. Often this is a parent, sibling, or other relative, but it may also be a friend, boyfriend, or girlfriend. It may include a previous placement resource, such as a former foster parent, or a person with whom the youth believes he or she has a relationship based on previous running episodes, such as a pimp or drug dealer.

- Some young people leave care without a destination in mind. They run, either alone or in the company of other youth, to escape their current placement, to seek freedom from the care and custody of adults in general or from the child welfare agency, to escape from bullying by other youth, to experience what they see as the excitement of life on their own, or as part of an overall pattern of risk taking. They may run voluntarily or be pressured or coerced into running by other youth or adults with whom they have a relationship.

- Some youth begin running before they enter care and continue to run as part of an established pattern. For these young people, running may not be about placement, but serves as a coping mechanism.

- The Florida Department of Law Enforcement and Florida Department of Children and Families (2002) have some evidence that some 16- and 17-year-old youth run as a first step toward establishing a life independent of the supervision of the agency.

Ascertaining into which category a runaway falls is an important part of determining every aspect of the child welfare agency's practice, from prevention through response, recovery, resolution, and ongoing planning. It also affects the response of the law enforcement agency charged with the investigation of the episode and recovery of the missing child.

Risks Faced by Runaways

Young people who run away, and especially those who run without a destination, are at heightened risk of both immediate and long-term harm. Without a known source of basic needs such as shelter, food, and clothing, the child may resort to stealing, drug dealing, prostitution, or other illegal and risky activities to support himself or herself, or may become a victim of violent acts, including sexual exploitation.

Children who remain missing for an extended period of time become disconnected from the educational system, health care, and housing. They set themselves up for negative outcomes, including dropping out of school, unemployment, homelessness, substance abuse, malnutrition, sexually transmitted diseases (including HIV/AIDS), and pregnancy.

The level of risk faced by any individual child depends on a number of factors, including the child's age and developmental level, previous history of victimization, and emotional and behavioral functioning, as well as the supports and dangers in the community.

Children Who Are Abducted

A child is considered abducted if someone without legal authority or permission of the custodian takes the child or fails to return the child at an agreed-on time. Abduction may be by a family or nonfamily member.

Children Abducted by Family Members or Other Caregivers

In a family abduction, a child is taken or not returned by a family member in violation of a court order, visitation agreement, or other legitimate custodial right. This may include children abducted by birthparents or kinship caregivers who disagree with the court's or agency's decision to reunify or change placements for another reason. Unless specific circumstances indicate that the child is in danger of abduction by a nonfamily member, such cases should be treated as family abductions, as the latter are significantly more prevalent.

Law enforcement personnel are familiar with cases in which children are abducted by family members, often in families undergoing a custody dispute, when one parent abducts the child from the custody of the other. When children are in the custody of a child welfare agency, however, all partners in the effort to locate and return the child must understand some distinctions:

- Most children in out-of-home care have been abused or neglected and removed from their parents' care to ensure their safety. Abduction by birthparents places children back in the care of the parents who maltreated them. In fact, children who alleged parental maltreatment and are abducted from care may be at heightened risk of maltreatment by parents who blame the child for the removal.

- When placement is not voluntary, family abduction from out-of-home care is in violation of a court order, because the court places children in out-of-home care.

- The legal custodian of the child is the child welfare agency, not the kinship family, foster family, group home, or residential facility in which the child is living.

- Substitute caregivers may have complex relationships with birthfamilies. Abduction scenarios include kinship caregivers assisting the birthparent in taking the child, and custody battles between the relative and the parent, particularly when substance abuse is involved or when maternal and paternal kin are in disagreement over the best interests of the child.

Children Abducted by Nonfamily Members

In a nonfamily abduction, a child is taken or not returned by a nonfamily member who does not have the lawful authority or permission of the child's legal custodian to do so. Nonfamily abduction includes:

- an episode in which a nonfamily member takes a child by the use of physical force or threat of bodily harm or detains the child for a substantial period of time (at least one hour) in an isolated place by the use of physical force or threat of bodily harm without lawful authority or permission of the caregiver;

- an episode in which a child younger than 15 or mentally incompetent, without lawful authority or permission of the caregiver, is taken or detained or voluntarily accompanies a nonfamily member, who conceals the child's whereabouts, demands ransom, or expresses the intention to keep the child permanently; or

- a stereotypical kidnapping, in which a child is taken by a stranger or slight acquaintance, transported 50 or more miles, detained overnight, held for ransom or with the intent to keep the child permanently, or killed. (Finkelhor et al., 2003)

Children Who Are "Lost" in Care

A child is considered lost if his or her whereabouts are unknown to the agency *and* this status is due to the inattentiveness of the agency. A child who is lost may be a runaway or may have been abducted, and his or her whereabouts are unknown to either the agency or the caregiver. Cases may also exist in which a caregiver is aware of the child's location, but the agency is not. This may be due to circumstances including:

- the caregiver has turned the physical custody of the child over to a third party without the knowledge or approval of the agency,

- the caregiver has failed to report that a child has run away or been abducted, or

- the agency has failed to maintain accurate, up-to-date records of the child's whereabouts and or to conduct face-to-face visits with the child and his or her caregivers.

Summary

The response to episodes of children missing from out-of-home care must be a joint effort between child welfare and law enforcement agencies. To facilitate that partnership, it is essential that a shared set of definitions be used to enable staff to communicate effectively.

In addition to shared definitions, partnering agencies need a common understanding of issues that make instances of children missing from out-of-home care different from instances in which children are missing from the care of their birthfamilies.

Both child welfare and law enforcement agencies can benefit from an understanding of the reasons children go missing from foster homes, group homes, and residential placements. This knowledge can help agencies develop practices and programs that prevent the occurrence of missing-from-care episodes by treating both the systemic and individual causes, enhancing investigative strategies and reducing recovery times, and implementing improved practices in the resolution of missing episodes.

When children in care do run away, they face the same risks as children who run from their families. Because many of them have histories of maltreatment and have experienced a breach of trust with adults in their lives, however, their emotional vulnerabilities and behavioral challenges pose a higher level of risk for some types of violence and exploitation, as well as for long-term disconnection from support, educational, and health systems.

Family abductions from out-of-home care may be different from those in which children are in the custody of birthparents because the state is the legal custodian of the child and because of the complex or strained relationships that can exist between birthfamilies and foster and kinship families. Child welfare agencies can contribute to law enforcement personnel's understanding of the complex family dynamics that may be different from those to which they are accustomed and that justify a higher level of concern.

The next chapter addresses critical issues in the management and administration of child welfare agencies that affect all aspects of missing-from-care cases, from prevention through return and resolution. It is through top-down agency values and policies as well as bottom-up procedures and practices that the agency demonstrates and carries out its commitment to maintaining children safely in its care.

CHAPTER 2

The Child Welfare Agency: Critical Issues in Management and Administration

Those who work with children in care must proactively work to prevent missing-from-care episodes, rather than merely reacting once a child has gone missing. The most effective way for agencies to prevent such episodes is to create an agencywide preventive approach based on the development and implementation of and support for quality practices and programs. In addition, successful prevention efforts are built on:

- the sound administration of child abuse and neglect prevention programs, as well as foster and residential care programs;

- quality supervision;

- effective training; and

- frequent contacts between workers and caregivers, workers and children in care, and children and their birthfamilies and other relatives.

Guidance for managing and administering these programs is provided in CWLA's *Standards of Excellence* in the areas of services for abused and neglected children and their families (1999b), family foster care services (1995), kinship care services (1999a), residential services (2004b), and transition, independent living, and self-sufficiency services (2005). Care for a child may be complicated by the involvement of both private and public foster homes and residential settings. A comprehensive prevention plan will ensure communication between private and public child welfare agencies and a comprehensive and dynamic data system.

Once a child is missing, the agency must be prepared to work in partnership with law enforcement agencies to respond to information requests from family members, caregivers, the general public, and the media; provide explanations for past actions and failures to courts, legislators, and policymakers; and remediate the situation and locate the child.

This chapter addresses critical issues for child welfare agencies to consider in their policies and practices. These policies and practices, in turn, must be supported by appropriate agency values and beliefs at all levels.

The child welfare agency's values, practices, and policies:

- provide a framework for the agency's efforts toward achieving positive outcomes for the children and families it serves;

- contribute to the prevention of missing-from-care episodes by responding to the needs of each child in out-of-home care and his or her family to ensure safety, permanency, and well-being for all children;

- reduce the time it takes to identify the location of missing children and return them safely to care; and

- contribute to a growing body of knowledge about missing children that enables the field to make continuous quality improvements in practices and policies as well as in the articulation and implementation of the value system on which they are based.

The Legal Framework

Legislation provides a foundation, context, and stimulus for the provision of child welfare services. Selected statutes—notably Title IV-E of the Social Security Act, the Personal Responsibility and Work Opportunities Reconciliation Act of 1996, and ASFA—address various aspects of out-of-home care that are related to issues involving children missing from care, but none contain specific provisions that speak specifically to the prevention of, response to, or resolution of missing episodes. CAPTA and the Keeping Children and Families Safe Act of 2003, which amended CAPTA, are concerned with the prevention and treatment of child abuse and neglect and encourage partnerships between child welfare agencies and other systems, including law enforcement, in those efforts, but do not address the issue of children missing from care.

The provisions of these laws, as well as others, including the Indian Child Welfare Act of 1978 and the Multi-Ethnic Placement Act of 1994, intersect with practice involving missing from care in such areas as safety and protection of children; recruitment, retention, and preparation of resource families to care for children in need of placement; selection of placement for each individual child; and the duty to provide permanency and maximize well-being for all children. Good practice in these areas plays an important role in the prevention of episodes in the first place and in their satisfactory resolution should such episodes occur.

The overarching philosophical tenet of ASFA—that the health and safety of children is the paramount concern that must guide all child welfare decisionmaking and service delivery—is the driving force behind the development of these guidelines.

Key Issues in Child Welfare Policy and Practice

Child welfare agencies must establish and implement policies and practices that maximize the safety of the children they serve, whether these children reside with birthfamilies, foster families, kinship caregivers, or adoptive families, or live in group care. A systematic review and examination of existing agency policies and practices is required to ensure that the outcomes achieved are those that are desired and that such policies and practices do not contribute, directly or indirectly, to the absences of children in the custody of the child welfare agency.

Systemic Issues Related to Runaways

Children who run from care may do so for child-specific or system-specific reasons.* System-specific reasons include lack of sufficient placement resources to meet the needs of the children needing care, inadequate staffing, inadequate training of staff or foster parents, inadequate monitoring of placements, and cultures (in the sense of atmosphere or environment) in homes or facilities that enable or encourage running episodes (Ross, 2001; Social Exclusion Unit, 2002; Wade & Biehal, 1998). Agencies must address those systemic issues that lead to an increased incidence of running away by:

- recruiting, training, and retaining a sufficient pool of competent foster parents who reflect the ethnic and racial diversity of children in the jurisdiction for whom foster homes are needed;

---

* Child-specific issues are addressed in Chapter 4, Prevention: Keeping Children and Youth Safely in Care.

- recruiting, training, and retaining a sufficient and competent workforce and maintaining caseload standards that permit workers to perform the duties necessary to achieve successful outcomes;

- providing staff and foster families with training and support to meet the needs of the children in care in ways that are safe, nurturing, consistent, and respectful of children's cultural, racial, ethnic, linguistic, and religious or spiritual backgrounds and sexual orientation;

- engaging in agencywide practices that are family centered, child focused and strengths based;

- including youth, birthparents, extended family, tribal members, and caregivers in all decisionmaking processes as appropriate;

- collecting data that enable the agency to determine prevalence and incidence of runaways at both state and local levels;

- examining the structure and operation of foster and group homes, residential facilities, or agencies that display higher rates of runaways; and

- implementing remedial actions, if necessary, to correct the structural and operational deficiencies that cause or contribute to running behavior of children in their care.

Systemic Issues Related to Abduction by Family Members

Of the entire population of children who go missing from care, those who are abducted by family members represent a small percentage of the whole. Available data do not permit an accurate estimate of the number of children who are abducted from care by family members. Practice wisdom, combined with limited research, indicates that between 5% and 15% of children missing from care have been abducted by family members (Florida Department of Law Enforcement & Florida Department of Children and Families, 2002; Hammer et al., 2002). The incidence of these episodes, whatever its exact proportion, can be decreased by:

- including birthparents, extended families, and foster parents as valued members of the service and permanency planning teams;

- maintaining connections between children and their families throughout placement;

- fostering communication between birth- and foster families;

- conducting safety and risk assessments that include consideration of parental behaviors that may be warning signs of potential abduction;

- developing and implementing visitation policies that build on safety and risk assessments and maximize child safety; and

- structuring supervised visitation when appropriate to continue and refine identification of potential risk.

Systemic Issues Related to Children "Lost" in Care

Child welfare agencies have come under fire in recent years for losing track of children in their custody. These include children who have run away or been abducted as well as those who may be in a placement but whose whereabouts are unknown due to failure to keep accurate records or provide adequate services to the child and the foster family or facility. No valid estimates exist for what percentage of children may fall into this category.

The agency must address the following issues to ensure that children are, to the greatest extent possible, not "lost" in care, and to minimize the trauma and effect on children, families, the community, and the agency when such incidents do occur:

- **Accountability and liability of the child welfare agency.** Agencies must accept full responsibility for the care of children who have been removed from their families and exercise ever-present diligence for the ongoing safety needs of these children.

- **Accurate record keeping and regular monitoring of placements.** Agencies must maintain current electronic or paper records of all children in their care, be able to access information about each child's location promptly, and use that information to monitor the location of the children through regular face-to-face contacts.

- **Systemwide identification of issues that are potential risks for children to be lost or forgotten in care.** Certain circumstances may heighten the risk to children of becoming lost or forgotten in care. Examples include workers with low rates of visits to children in care, limited communication about child moves between private and public agencies, falsification of records, children placed out of state, and children with specific characteristics.

- **Periodic census of all children in the custody of the agency.** A periodic census ensures that data are accurate, provides verification of placement, and identifies systemwide risks for losing children.

- **Involvement of multiple parties in an emotionally challenging experience.** The process and procedures that are established to identify the location of missing children must be responsive to all the parties involved—children, birthfamilies, foster families, and child welfare staff. Agencies must provide all parties with timely, relevant information while simultaneously not compromising the integrity of the search and ability to recover the child.

- **Response to the media and the public.** Agencies must be prepared to respond to media and community demands for information about the status of children in their care with a protocol that details how, when, what, and with whom information should be shared to facilitate the recovery of children. Such releases of information should comply with the confidentiality and privacy protections of children and their families as detailed in federal and state statutes and policies.

Agencies may wish to establish a dedicated missing child unit. Those who staff such a unit should be prepared with the knowledge, training, and expertise necessary to work closely with law enforcement personnel to locate missing children. In addition, these staff might be responsible for developing processes, establishing liaisons, monitoring protocols, and conducting staff training throughout the agency.

Training

Training of members of the planning and service team is an essential aspect of the child welfare agency's efforts to prevent missing episodes. The agency has a responsibility to:

- prepare its staff, foster parents, and other service providers with the knowledge and skills they need to understand child and family issues that lead to missing episodes;

- recognize warning signs and respond appropriately to them;

- implement agency policies and practices that lessen the likelihood of children going missing;

- promptly initiate recovery efforts when children do go missing; and

- decrease trauma and increase responsiveness to children's needs on their return.

Training alone is not sufficient to ensure that workers implement the practices that are taught. Agencies should supplement training courses with other methods of information sharing and knowledge and skill development, such as distribution of relevant materials, periodic reminders and review, supervision, case review, and opportunities to practice skills used infrequently.

Agency staff, foster parents, and other service providers should all receive training in the knowledge and skills displayed in Table 1.

Caseworkers

Agencies should identify core competencies that all child welfare workers responsible for working with children in care, their families, and foster families must master as part of preservice training. In addition, agencies should identify advanced and specialized competencies to be addressed in ongoing inservice training for each category of worker employed by them. Assignment of cases and tasks to workers should take into consideration the training they have received and the level of competency they have attained.

Caseworkers should receive training in the knowledge and skills displayed in Table 1, as well as the knowledge and skills set forth below that focus specifically on the prevention of children missing in care:

- soliciting the views of the birthparents and the child, as appropriate, when determining placement selection;

- making appropriate placements based on the foster family's capacity to meet the unique needs of the child;

- placing children in the least restrictive, most family-like, and most appropriate setting available, consistent with the child's best interests and special needs;

- maintaining stability of the placement based on the knowledge of the impact of placement on children, birthfamilies, and foster families;

Table 1. Knowledge and Skills for Caseworkers, Supervisors, and Foster Parents that Contribute to the Prevention of Missing Episodes

Knowledge	Skills
• Importance and dynamics of collaboration and teaming.	• Serve as a partner on a collaborative child welfare team.
• Importance of involvement of birthparents, youth in care, and foster parents in assessment, service planning, and problem resolution.	• Participate in inclusive planning and problem resolution.
• Potential effects of placement on children, birthfamilies, and foster families, including effects of separation and loss on children's mental health status and behaviors.	• Help children confront and cope with trauma related to removal from birthfamilies. • Include children, whenever appropriate and possible, in making decisions that affect them. • Help birthfamilies confront and cope with trauma related to removal of their children. • Recognize unique needs of children in care. • Employ effective strategies to address those needs.
• Normal child and adolescent development issues and ways in which both maltreatment and placement in out-of-home care affect development.	• Recognize the emotional and behavioral developmental levels of children, regardless of age. • Help children confront and cope with issues of living in out-of-home care in ways that are developmentally appropriate. • Employ effective strategies to address behavioral and emotional challenges, including those resulting from separation and loss and the trauma of placement.
• Need for open communication with children in placement.	• Establish positive relationships and develop patterns of open communication with children and youth in care. • Establish a supportive relationship with children based on trust and mutual respect.
• Importance of parent/child visitation and sibling visitation in maintaining continuity and culture, contributing to child well-being, and achieving permanence.	• Facilitate regular visitation with birthparents, siblings, and other relatives that ensures safety. • Help children and their families make progress toward permanency goals.
• Process and effect of a youth's transition to interdependent living.	• Work with other professionals to assess the young person's ability and willingness to live interdependently. • Participate in developing and implementing a plan to prepare a young person for interdependent living. • Use a variety of methods to help youth gain the competencies essential for interdependent living.
• Risk and safety factors for children residing in out-of-home care.	• Use observation, assessment, interviewing, and consultation with the child, professionals, and others involved in the child's life to identify risk and safety factors.

- advocating for the best interests of the child with other service agencies; and

- conducting ongoing safety and risk assessments at relevant decision points throughout the life of the case.

Supervisors

Supervisors should be able to support, assist, inform, and instruct their workers. Agencies should expect supervisors to be proficient in the core competencies expected of child welfare workers under their supervision, as well as in supervisory competencies necessary to support workers, promote growth on the job, ensure that workers meet administrative and legal responsibilities, determine that staff meet performance standards, and provide individualized training (CWLA, 1995).

Training must provide supervisors with the knowledge of and skills needed for oversight of daily casework, including, but not limited to:

- overseeing workers' periodic, quality visitation with the child in care;

- overseeing case documentation of the child's status in placement;

- ensuring that regular assessments of safety threats and risk factors that may pose potential flight risks occur;

- identifying services necessary to reduce risks of flight; and

- handling expeditious and appropriate responses to situations in which the child's placement may result in the child's absence.

Foster Parents

Foster parents should be trained so that they acquire the necessary values, knowledge, and skills to effectively perform their responsibilities to meet the needs of children and the requirements of the agency. Agencies should identify core competencies that should be attained by all foster parents as part of preservice training as well as advanced and specialized competencies to be addressed in ongoing inservice training. Foster parents should receive training in the knowledge and skills displayed in Table 1. Additional foster parent competencies that are specific to the prevention and resolution of missing from out-of-home care episodes include:

- the importance of promoting a child's positive sense of identity, history, culture, and values to help develop self-esteem;

- the importance of creating a supportive and accepting family environment and providing unconditional positive support; and

- who to contact and what actions to take if a child in the foster parent's care goes missing.

To safeguard children in their care, foster parents must have an awareness of risks associated with running away and strategies to prevent both running and abduction. The child welfare agency must offer foster parents the support, supervision, and training to develop skills to enable them to deter children from unauthorized absences and must provide the foster parents with the understanding and competence to follow prescribed agency procedures when children leave care without permission.

Staff

Staff at group homes and residential care facilities should be trained so that they acquire the necessary values, knowledge, and skills to effectively perform their job responsibilities. Children in group and residential settings are more likely than children in family homes to run away from care (Courtney & Wong, 1996; Ross, 2001) and are more likely to run without a destination in mind (Biehal & Wade, 1999). Because children in residential care are at a higher risk for running away and the attendant dangers associated with such episodes, staff should receive specialized training in:

- understanding why children and youth run from placements, recognizing behavioral and emotional indicators that a child may be at increased risk of running, and taking appropriate actions to prevent running episodes, which might include addressing child-specific or systemic reasons for running or bringing them to the attention of supervisory staff;

- developing a relationship of trust with the child or youth or encouraging such a relationship with another adult;

- encouraging visits with the child's family and siblings;

- ensuring that children are receiving the services called for in their service plans, such as keeping appointments with mental health professionals;

- providing education on the risks associated with running; and

- being watchful of situations such as youth being bullied by other children.

Staff at group homes and residential care facilities should all receive training in the knowledge and skills displayed in Table 1. Because such staff fill the roles of foster parents for children in their care, they should be trained to achieve the same competencies needed by foster parents. In addition, they should possess skills in:*

- objectively assessing children and families, identifying strengths and needs, and making sound decisions based on the information gathered;

- engaging children and families in addressing immediate and long-term needs for safety and well-being;

- interacting with children, youth, and families in a culturally responsive manner;

- assessing the risk and safety factors in the residential setting and taking decisive action when additional protection is needed;

- establishing rapport with children and motivating them toward individual changes;

- using authority constructively to protect children and support families;

- working under stress and effectively responding to crises that occur in a variety of settings; and

- seeking and using consultation and supervision as needed.

Foster Parent Recruitment and Retention

Across the country, agencies have a shortage of foster homes in general and of families that meet the unique needs of children served by the child welfare system. These shortages can lead to poor placement matches, which may increase the risk of children running from care as well as multiple placement moves and placement in settings other than family foster homes.

Agencies responsible for placing children in out-of-home care have a primary responsibility to conduct ongoing, diligent recruitment campaigns that will enable them to maintain an adequate pool of competent foster parents who:

---

* These skills are identified in CWLA's *Standards of Excellence for Residential Services* (2004b). Only those skills relevant to the prevention of and response to missing episodes are included.

- reflect the ethnic and racial diversity of children in the state for whom foster and adoptive homes are needed;

- live in the neighborhoods from which the children come;

- have a demonstrated knowledge of, commitment to, and concern for children; and

- can parent children with the unique needs, characteristics, and issues represented in the population needing care.

Having such a pool of foster parents available at all times enables the agency to make the best possible placement choices, taking into account the wishes, needs, and best interests of the child and his or her birthfamily as well as the ability of the foster parents to meet those needs.

Recruitment is only the first step in the agency's responsibility for maintaining an adequate pool of competent foster families. Training, discussed previously, is necessary to prepare foster parents for their roles and to facilitate the ongoing development of knowledge and skills to help foster parents work effectively with the children in their care as well as their families. Agencies must also provide other supports to retain foster parents on a long-term basis. These supports include, but are not limited to, adequate compensation, respite, child care, mentoring, in-home crisis or stabilization services, and peer support groups. Above all, agencies must create and display an organizational climate that incorporates and reinforces respect for foster parents in all practices, including accessibility to and contact with caseworkers based on the foster family's need for support and monitoring.

Record Keeping

Accurate and up-to-date records are essential to knowing the whereabouts of children in the agency's care, understanding each child's history and current status, planning for his or her future, and knowing whether current or prior placements have been responsive to the child's needs. CWLA's *Standards of Excellence for Family Foster Care Services* (1995) suggests that service records be retained for 50 years from the time of the child's discharge from the agency. Using this as a guidepost, child welfare agencies should establish and adhere to their own policies regarding the retention of records.

Case Files

Case files, which may be paper or electronic, should include information that can assist in locating and properly identifying a missing child as well as information that enables the agency to contact family members promptly. Case files should include the following information, which should be updated promptly whenever a change occurs:

- child's names and nicknames;
- child's address;
- child's telephone numbers;
- child's e-mail address;
- names, addresses, telephone numbers, and e-mail addresses for both parents as well as maternal and paternal relatives, and siblings;
- names, addresses, telephone numbers, and e-mail addresses for friends or other people the child may have run away with or to in the past;
- prior addresses of parents, relatives, and siblings;
- a digital photograph of the child, updated every six months until the child is 6 years old and at least annually after that, with additional updates if there are obvious changes in appearance;
- a description of the child, including height, weight, hair, eye, and skin color, and other identifying marks, updated every six months until the child is 6 years old and at least annually after that, with additional updates if there are obvious changes in appearance;
- child's fingerprints;
- child's dental records;
- child's Social Security number;
- child's birth certificate; and
- reports of worker contacts with the child.

Management Information Systems

Quality management information systems (MIS) are essential to agency infrastructure in all aspects of operation, and particularly in the prevention of as well as intervention with children missing from care. The child welfare agency has a responsibility to record and update the agency's information system with accurate data regarding the child's whereabouts and current status.

An electronic information system should capture and maintain current information about the child, including identifying and contact information, and should be updated promptly whenever a change occurs. Reports should be generated regularly that enable the agency to identify children who are not being visited by a caseworker at appropriate intervals and those for whom conflicting data may be an indication that the child is not located at his or her approved placement. The MIS should be able to track the whereabouts of children in both public and private child care facilities.

In addition, the data system should provide a way to record information that can be used to contribute to the body of knowledge about missing children. This should include the following information regarding missing episodes:

- whether the child is missing or has returned;

- length of time missing;

- suspected type of missing episode (runaway or abduction);

- determined type of missing episode (runaway or abduction) once the child has returned;

- efforts made to locate the child;

- location of the child when found, or during missing episode; and

- reason for running or other absence.

To the extent possible, the agency MIS should have the capacity to provide the information needed by law enforcement systems. When an automatic interface is not possible, the next best alternative is amanual interface and a procedure for frequent and regular updates.

Child welfare agencies should also work to develop and maintain systems that are capable of interfacing with those of child welfare agencies in other states, facilitating the sharing of information when children go missing across state lines.

Agencies without data collection or an MIS currently in place, or those with systems that do not capture the full range of information needed to record and track missing episodes, should work to develop and implement such systems. Child welfare agencies may institute procedures to collect data regarding children missing from care using computer spreadsheets or databases that are capable of maintaining statistical information and producing reports at the local, if not county- or statewide, level. While doing so, the child welfare agency should consider working with the local law enforcement agency to assist in creating a system that will generate qualitative and quantitative reports on children missing from the agency's care using the local law enforcement agency's missing children's database, state clearinghouse, or NCIC system.

Agencywide Census of Children in Care

Child welfare agencies can take a proactive approach to verifying the safety and placement of all children in their care by conducting an agencywide annual census. At minimum, such a census should consist of a personal verification that all children in out-of-home care are physically located in their court-ordered placement. The census, which can be conducted by agency staff, community partners, or volunteers such as students of social work, can also be used to gather other information and data such as permanency and well-being indicators; strengths, challenges, and needs of children in care, their families, and their caregivers; gaps in the service array; and training needs. Such a census should also be targeted to assess the quality of the system and identify potential risks for losing children in care.

Children Who Age Out While Missing

Some percentage of children who go missing from care reach the age at which they would ordinarily be emancipated from the custody of the child welfare agency or the age they become ineligible for services (e.g., education, health, and housing assistance) related to the process of attaining full independence. If such young people are removed from the data system but later located or recovered by a law enforcement agency, the agency may have no way to identify them. To ensure that the child's identity can be determined under such circumstances and even after he or she has aged out of care, child welfare agencies should collaborate with the court and law enforcement agencies to develop protocols enabling them to discharge the missing young person from the care of the agency at an appropriate age while still maintaining records that will permit prompt and accurate identification if he or she is located.

Interjurisdictional Issues

Children may be placed across agency, county, or state lines for a number of reasons, including enabling a relative to provide foster care, facilitating placement with a foster family or preadoptive family able to meet a child's unique needs, or securing therapeutic or treatment services in a group home or residential facility with services not available in the placing agency's jurisdiction. When this occurs, both the sending agency or state and the receiving agency or state should accept responsibility for the safety of the child.

Although the Interstate Compact on the Placement of Children provides that the sending agency retains jurisdiction over the child,* it also allows the sender to "enter into an agreement with an authorized public or private agency in the receiving state providing for the performance of one or more services in respect of such case by the latter as agent for the sending agency" (Article V. [a]). To ensure the best interests of children placed across state lines, agencies should develop agreements that address issues relevant to the prevention, recovery, and return of children missing from care. These include the following:

- Children should receive regular, meaningful visits from caseworkers in the jurisdiction in which they reside, and the receiving agency should share documentation of such visits with the sending agency. The agency with custody of the child must assume responsibility for that child's safety, permanency, and well-being, and should ensure that visits to the child occur.

- Both agencies should maintain adequate records about the child's location and placement, and update one another whenever a change is made.

- Both agencies should maintain up-to-date case files including current photographs, fingerprints, and other identifying information that could be used to locate the child if he or she went missing.

Much like other interagency agreements, the purpose, terms, and methods for monitoring, evaluating, and renewing such agreements should be specified in writing.

Confidentiality and the Need to Share Information

The rights to confidentiality and privacy protections are fundamental tenets of child welfare practice, but the safety of children in care and the safe return of those missing from care may depend on the ability and willingness of child welfare agencies to share information with foster parents, law enforcement

---

* At the time of this writing, revisions to the Interstate Compact on the Placement of Children are under consideration; the government has not formally adopted new provisions.

agencies, community partners, and in some cases the media and the general public. Agency policy should permit the sharing of information vital to the safe return of a missing child or protection of a child about whom someone has made a threat of abduction. Agencies should inform and encourage caseworkers and other agency staff to share such information when requested. Child welfare agency policy should clearly state what information can be shared, with whom, and for what purposes.

Working with Law Enforcement

Law enforcement agencies need swift access to child welfare agency records at the beginning of their investigation of a child missing from care. The following policies and practices can facilitate the timely sharing of necessary information:

- A memorandum of understanding (MOU) between the agencies should clearly articulate the type of information law enforcement personnel consider necessary to the conduct of an investigation as well as the categories of information the child welfare agency is permitted to share.

- Child welfare agencies should designate an individual in the agency to receive all requests for information concerning missing children. That person should make case-by-case determinations regarding the specific case file information to be shared with the law enforcement agency, using published agency policy and criteria as essential guidelines.

- Procedures in the child welfare agency about the routing of such information requests to the designated individual should be clear to all staff from whom it may be requested, including caseworkers, supervisors, and staff responsible for receiving incoming telephone calls.

Media Issues

Cases in which children are missing from care may attract the attention of local media and, in high-profile cases, national media. Child welfare agencies should be prepared to handle such requests by proactively preparing a plan that enables appropriate personnel to control the flow of information to the media, share information that may be helpful to locating the missing child, and maintain the confidentiality of the child and family to the extent possible.

- **Point of Contact:** One person should be the designated spokesperson for the agency, and all communication with the media should be through that individual. The spokesperson must be given ready access to all relevant parties, including the leaders and decision-makers in both child welfare and law enforcement agencies.

- **Letters of Understanding:** Child welfare agencies may consider the development of a letter of understanding that would authorize the state clearinghouses (see p. 32) to create flyers of missing children that would be disseminated to NCMEC for publication on its website and further distribution to the general public.

- **Case-Specific Information:** The type of information about a missing child that can be shared with the media will depend on the circumstances of the particular case as well as state-specific statutes and policies. In most instances, shared information should be limited to that which can help in the location and recovery of the child, such as name, age, description, circumstances of disappearance, and so forth. Although the general plan can cover broad categories of information, one person should be designated to make determinations about specific cases. This individual should have a comprehensive understanding of issues related to agency liability and client confidentiality in addition to other legal considerations. This individual may also be designated to determine what information the agency should share with law enforcement personnel.

- **Other Information to Be Shared:** In the course of covering a missing child case, media may request additional information, including statistics about other children missing from care, both locally and nationally. The agency plan should include a fact sheet, updated at least annually, with information responsive to such media requests.

- **Positive Messaging:** Rather than reacting to negative charges from the community or the media, the agency should be prepared to take responsibility when it is warranted, commit to change when necessary, and meet the media with a positive message that focuses on locating the missing child and ensuring the ongoing safety and well-being of all children in the care and custody of the agency.

Coordination with Community Partners

All children, including those in out-of-home care, are at reduced risk for going missing when community systems work together to ensure child safety, provide developmentally appropriate safety education to children, respond to and reduce risks in the community, and form partnerships for reducing the possibility of running or abduction for those children at increased risk.

Child welfare and law enforcement agencies should work with schools and other community partners to ensure that all children are enrolled in school- or community-based child safety education programs, are educated about the risks of running away, and have access to information on both maintaining safety and accessing confidential assistance and communication services if they do run. Child welfare agencies should also engage partners in the health, mental health, and education systems; the courts; and other community service providers, such as runaway and shelter programs, in the development of a comprehensive system of care that addresses the safety, permanency, and well-being of all children in the community.

Agencies should educate physical and mental health care providers, school personnel, and other community resources that work with children, such as clergy and sports associations, about the early warning signs that may precede runaway episodes as well as the risks of running for children and youth. Joint training by child welfare and law enforcement staff on these issues can provide all community partners with a shared understanding of and commitment to prevention.

A Comprehensive Agency Plan

The child welfare agency can approach the issue of children missing from care in a proactive manner by preparing a comprehensive plan that includes both systemwide activities and processes and individual responsibilities of staff, supervisors, and administrators. The plan should be based on current knowledge about the issue of children missing from care, relevant research findings, and existing best practices. The agency plan should include sections on:

- MOUs with law enforcement or other agencies;
- relevant statutory and policy provisions;
- confidentiality and information sharing;

- record keeping, data collection, and MIS;

- interjurisdictional monitoring of children;

- training requisites for personnel;

- protocols for the response to and investigation, recovery, return, and debriefing of missing children; and

- oversight and evaluation of the plan.

Summary

Federal legislation—most notably, ASFA—demands that the child welfare agency be responsible for ensuring the safety of children in out-of-home care. Agency policies and practices that contribute to the prevention of missing episodes as well as those that facilitate the expeditious return of children who have gone missing are essential components of that commitment to safety.

Agencies must address systemic issues that contribute to missing-from-care episodes, including those known to increase the likelihood that children and youth will run from foster homes or other placements and those that may encourage birthparents or other relatives to attempt to abduct children from care. Agencies can reduce the likelihood of both running and family abduction by (a) improving agency practice in the recruitment, retention, and support of foster parents; (b) training foster parents and child welfare staff; and (c) improving relationships between birthfamilies and foster families. Agencies have a responsibility to select placements that meet the unique needs of children in their care. They must keep accurate and current records on all children in care to ensure that children are not lost and to facilitate the speedy location and recovery of children who do go missing.

Agencies should take a proactive approach to the issue of missing children by preparing a plan that details intra- and interagency policy and procedures on issues including, but not limited to, partnership with law enforcement and other community agencies, confidentiality and information sharing, media contact, and staff protocols for the prevention of, response to, return of, and recovery of missing children.

CHAPTER 3

The Law Enforcement Agency: An Essential Partnership

The primary goal of both law enforcement and child welfare agencies in cases of children missing from care is the safe return of children to the adults responsible for their care. This is the foundation of their partnership. This chapter provides an overview of the legal framework that shapes the law enforcement response to missing-from-care episodes, the responsibilities of law enforcement agencies, and the skills and tools they bring to the investigation of children who go missing. The chapter also focuses on issues that both law enforcement and child welfare agencies must address to maximize their collaborative efforts to locate and return missing children.

The Legal Framework

Federal legislation in the areas of juvenile justice and law enforcement addresses children who are missing; no specific provisions exist regarding youth in out-of-home care. The provisions of these statutes provide a framework for the investigative work of law enforcement agencies and promote the development of reporting and investigative tools that guide law enforcement agencies.

- The Runaway and Homeless Youth Act established the National Runaway Switchboard to enable runaways to communicate with their families as well as to provide nonsecure facilities where youngsters in need can receive safe shelter, counseling, and education until an effective family reunion can be accomplished.

- The Parental Kidnapping Prevention Act of 1980 extended resources available to law enforcement in investigating cases of parental abduction.

- The Missing Children's Assistance Act of 1984 created a national toll-free number for reporting information about missing children and provides technical assistance to those seeking to locate them.

- The National Child Search Assistance Act of 1990 required that all law enforcement agencies must accept missing-child cases immediately, without a waiting period; must enter reports of missing children younger than 18 into the NCIC system; and must update identifying information in a timely manner.

- The Child Safety Act, a provision of the Violent Crime Control and Law Enforcement Act of 1994, provided for the establishment of supervised visitation centers to allow children at risk of harm from their parents to visit them in a safe environment.

- The Prosecutorial Remedies and Other Tools to End the Exploitation of Children Today Act of 2003 included provisions for

  — Suzanne's Law, which requires each federal, state, and local law enforcement agency to enter information about missing adults between the ages of 18 and 21 into the NCIC missing person database;

  — the establishment of procedures for handling a child missing or lost in a public building, known as a Code Adam alert; and

  — the enhancement of the "America's Missing: Broadcast Emergency Response (AMBER) Alert" plan. The act calls for the national coordination of state and local AMBER Alert plans and clearly defined activation criteria, such as sufficient descriptive information about the victim and abduction for law enforcement to issue an AMBER Alert to assist in the recovery of a child who is in imminent danger of serious bodily injury or death.

In addition to these federal laws, many states have legislatively mandated specific actions to be taken in missing child cases. MOUs between law enforcement and child welfare agencies should include information about any such laws and should be updated in accordance with the passage of new relevant legislative provisions.

Responsibilities of the Law Enforcement Agency

Law enforcement agencies are statutorily and ethically responsible for taking appropriate investigative action in all missing child cases, regardless of the circumstances under which the child is missing. This includes promptly entering information into the NCIC missing person files for all missing children as well as missing adults from ages 18 to 21. Waiting periods are prohibited under federal and state laws. Federal and state mandates for entering dental records, photographs, and other identifying information also apply.

The law enforcement agency must complete a missing-person report whenever a child welfare agency determines a child is missing from care. It should provide child welfare agencies with the necessary data elements to be captured for the detailed reporting of a missing child. It may be appropriate to provide blank copies of the missing-person report to child welfare representatives to help ensure that complete information is made available to investigating officers as quickly as possible.

Law enforcement agency policies and procedures must identify jurisdiction and response protocols. Law enforcement policies may require missing-child reports be made in the jurisdiction where the child was last seen. This does not, however, preclude collaboration with and possible transfer of the cases to the law enforcement agency having jurisdiction where the child resided prior to disappearing.

Resources and Services

The National Center for Missing & Exploited Children (NCMEC)

NCMEC is the congressionally mandated national resource center and clearinghouse dedicated to issues involving missing and sexually exploited children. It provides several resources.

- **Case Management and Technical Assistance.** Well-trained and experienced case managers who have had extensive law enforcement careers work with law enforcement and child welfare agencies and provide advice and assistance in collecting evidence, getting search warrants, interviewing victims, and conducting searches. They also provide assistance to family members.

- **Case Analysis.** NCMEC's Case Analysis and Support Division assesses leads and provides the most usable, relevant information possible to law enforcement agencies and state clearinghouses. Using NCMEC databases, external data sources, and geographic-information databases, analysts track leads, identify patterns between cases, and help coordinate investigations by linking cases together.

- **Imaging and Identification Services.** NCMEC provides computerized age progression of the photographs of long-term missing children, reconstruction of facial images from morgue photographs of unidentified deceased juveniles so posters may be made to assist in the child's identification, computer assistance in creating artist composites, assistance in identifying faces of children whose images are found in confiscated child pornography, and training in imaging applications and techniques.

- **Photo and Poster Distribution.** NCMEC maintains an up-to-date database of missing-children posters on the CompuServe® and state clearinghouse private, bulletin-board computer networks. NCMEC can broadcast fax posters and other case-related information to more than 26,000 law enforcement agencies throughout the nation. NCMEC also coordinates national media exposure of missing-children cases through its partnership with major television networks, leading nationwide publications, and major corporations.

- **Computer Networking.** Online services provide links with 50 state clearinghouses plus the District of Columbia and Puerto Rico, the U.S. Secret Service Forensic Services Division, the U.S. Department of State, the U.S. Immigration and Customs Enforcement, and other entities. This allows the instant transmission of missing children's images and information about these cases.

- **Training and Publications.** NCMEC provides training in all aspects of missing- and exploited-child cases. Courses range from regional, investigative training sessions to policy-development seminars. NCMEC also publishes a wealth of materials and is available to assist families as well as law enforcement and child welfare professionals.

State Clearinghouses

Every state has a missing-children clearinghouse, usually located in a state police or criminal justice agency. Although state clearinghouse capabilities vary, many provide investigative support services to law enforcement agencies, support and guidance to left-behind family members, and public education programs. All state clearinghouses work closely with NCMEC.

Key Issues in Partnerships with Law Enforcement Agencies

Child welfare staff and law enforcement personnel have a shared interest in the safe return of children missing from out-of-home care. When child welfare and law enforcement agencies work in partnership, they bring the expertise of both disciplines to the table, which can enhance both the investigative effort and the resolution of the episode. It is essential that both partners also bring a respect for the other's point of view and knowledge, an openness to different ways of working and thinking, and a willingness to work together in the best interest of the child who is missing.

Law enforcement and child welfare agencies lack a common frame of reference for the issues that make these cases different from those in which children are missing from their birthfamilies. Child welfare staff bring to the partnership a set of values, knowledge, and skills that focus on the safety, permanency, and well-being of children who have been removed from the care of their parents for reasons of abuse and neglect, and they dedicate much of their work to the relationships between children and birthfamilies, children and foster families or other caregivers, and birthfamilies and caregivers. They are trained in a strengths-based, family-centered perspective and approach, and make assessments based on their knowledge of a variety of topics, including family dynamics and child development.

For law enforcement personnel, the focus of their work is on the investigation necessary to locate and return the child safely to the care of the agency. Their efforts are dedicated to finding facts, collecting evidence, and upholding the law. Their knowledge of family dynamics may focus more on the specific circumstances, problems, and individual characteristics that may lead to abduction or runaway episodes.

Elements of Partnership

Substantive and ongoing collaboration between child welfare and law enforcement agencies is essential to provide an adequate and prompt response when children are missing. Agencies can enhance collaboration by gaining consensus about and adopting key definitional and procedural elements.

Shared Definitions. The need for clear, consistent definitions of *missing* in both statute and policy is essential to effective communication and coordination of efforts to locate children who are missing. Standardized definitions facilitate a more expeditious and appropriate response by all parties. Agency partners should establish mutually acceptable categories of absences within the framework of state statutes, each with its own level of risk and expected response as part of the framework of joint practice.

Joint Protocols for Response. A clear delineation of the shared and distinct roles and responsibilities of child welfare staff, law enforcement personnel, and other statutory and voluntary agencies that may be involved in the response to, investigation of, and recovery of children missing from care enhances recovery efforts, reduces confusion, shortens response time, and increases efficient use of personnel and other resources.

Cross-System Training. Child welfare and law enforcement agencies can benefit from joint training efforts that share specific information on agency and collaborative protocols for handling cases of children missing from care as well as the values and beliefs that shape each agency's policy and practice. By interacting with employees of other professions during training, child welfare and law enforcement personnel gain a better understanding of the specific problems and issues faced by their counterparts. Cross-systems training should include information about:

- child welfare agency policy on reporting missing children and law enforcement policy on accepting reports;
- information contained in NCIC, and state and local information systems employed by both agencies;
- procedures for investigating missing-children cases;
- tools available for use by both agencies; and
- communication and coordination between child welfare and law enforcement.

Shared Information Systems. The creation and maintenance of an integrated local information system is essential to meet the needs of frontline child welfare and law enforcement staff and facilitate cross-system information sharing and a coordinated response. Law enforcement agencies have used automated information sharing systems for decades. NCIC instituted the Missing Person File in 1975, enabling agencies nationwide to verify and access reports of missing children. In 1984, the Missing Children's Assistance Act required agencies to enter all missing-children cases into this file.

Confidentiality Protocols. Law enforcement agencies seek to gather as much information as possible to conduct investigations. Child welfare agencies operate under statutory and policy guidance that includes specific regulations concerning the types of information that they can disclose about children and families, and to whom. Protocols should clarify and streamline confidentiality requirements so that professionals, agencies, and jurisdictions can share pertinent information. Such protocols should also delineate what information agencies can and cannot share with caregivers and birthfamily members.

Jointly Prepared Procedures. Creating a joint framework for policy and procedure will provide informed, prepared, trained, and cohesive responses to adequately investigate a child missing from care case. Appendix A lists a variety of specific activities to consider.

Information Systems

Law enforcement agencies employ a number of tools for capturing, storing, and sharing information about missing children, including the NCIC database, state and local missing-children clearinghouses, the Federal Parent Locator Service, and agency proprietary databases. Some child welfare systems may collect the data elements necessary to conduct a missing-person search or investigation. It is important that child welfare and law enforcement agencies make inroads toward the identification and interface of common data elements, either manually or automatically, and work together to develop systems that:

- collect the data elements necessary to the conduct of a missing-person investigation,
- allow for immediate access when someone reports a missing child,
- can be easily and quickly updated to reflect new information, and
- automatically interface with one another.

Current state-of-the-art information technology enables a state child welfare agency to complete electronic input into its information system as well as the system maintained by the state's law enforcement agency. Local law enforcement agencies can provide guidance on the development of systems that interface with local, state, and federal databases, enabling child welfare agencies to overcome their own jurisdictional limits and expand searches and investigation beyond county or state boundaries.

The first 48 hours after a child goes missing are the most critical in locating and returning the child to safety. Law enforcement and child welfare agencies should jointly explore the use of the Internet, intra- and extranets, fax, telephone, e-mail, electronic data notification, and AMBER Alert systems to speed the effort to make information about missing children available to the agencies and, where appropriate, communities and media who can assist in finding those children.

Agencies should also undertake joint efforts to facilitate the exchange of information with child welfare and law enforcement agencies in other states when children cross state borders for placement.

MOUs

A well-written MOU can improve practice by providing written guidelines for roles and responsibilities of member agencies in investigations and other multidisciplinary functions, serving as a reference when questions arise about practice, establishing consistency, and reducing the need for on-the-spot decisionmaking by defining protocols in advance. The result is more effective prevention, faster response, greater efficiency, and reduced trauma for families and caregivers. An MOU between child welfare and law enforcement agencies on the subject of children missing from care should include, at a minimum, the information listed in Appendix B.

Summary

Law enforcement agencies operate pursuant to federal and state statutes that prescribe actions that they must take in response to reports of missing children. Child welfare agencies, working in partnership with law enforcement in these investigations, should be aware of the responsibilities of law enforcement agencies as well as the resources and services they can expect law enforcement to provide.

Partnerships between law enforcement and child welfare agencies must be marked by mutual respect for each other's viewpoints, knowledge, and skills. Agencies can pave the way toward effectively working in concert by paying attention to the details of the elements of the partnership, including shared definitions, joint protocols for response, cross-training, shared information systems, and confidentiality protocols.

Federal, state, and local information systems are key law enforcement tools in the recovery of missing children. Child welfare agencies should work closely with law enforcement in the development and implementation of systems that interface with and provide essential information to both agencies.

The completion of an MOU between the law enforcement and child welfare agencies ensures that roles and responsibilities are clearly defined for all phases of work with missing children, from prevention through return and resolution. Agencies that implement such a protocol will be able to respond more quickly and more effectively when children do go missing from out-of-home care.

CHAPTER 4

Prevention: Keeping Children and Youth Safely in Care

Child welfare practices that can reduce the incidence of missing from care episodes are generally those that adhere to the CWLA *Standards of Excellence for Family Foster Care Services* (1995) in the areas of assessment and service planning, placement, providing and monitoring services, and permanency planning, as well as community-based support for family foster care services. Those practices particularly relevant to the prevention of missing episodes will be discussed in this chapter.

The Prevention Team

Prevention of missing episodes is the duty of the entire team of individuals who are responsible for the child in out-of-home care. CWLA's *Standards of Excellence for Family Foster Care Services* (1995, p. 32) identify the following as potential participants in the assessment and service-planning team for family foster care:

- family foster care agency staff members and foster parents who work with the child;
- the public agency social worker who was involved in the referral and intake;
- parents, siblings, grandparents, godparents, and other significant family and kinship members;
- adoptive parents;
- the child, according to age and development;
- clergy;
- teachers;
- counselors or other professionals who have an important or potentially important relationship with the child; and
- court representatives.

Each of these parties may contribute information that can help the team assess the likelihood of the child running from any placement in general, and a specific placement in particular, about the potential risk of family abduction, and about the child's vulnerability to non–family member abduction. Any of these individuals may have knowledge about child risk and protective factors that may be important in the development of safety and risk assessments. In addition, they may be able to contribute information about the child's relationship with his or her parents and other family members, the child's and family's history and coping mechanisms, and the extent to which the child makes use of services and supports available to him or her in the family and the community. By listening to the input of all team members beginning with the initial assessment and continuing throughout the length of the placement, the agency can make the most accurate possible determination of the potential risk of the child leaving care without permission or of being abducted by a family member or non–family member. In addition, for all children, including those in the child welfare system, schools, law enforcement agencies, and other community partners who can develop and manage communitywide prevention programs should be considered part of the prevention team.

Preparation for Placement

For any child in out-of-home care, prevention begins prior to placement, with appropriate preparation of the child, the birthfamily, and the caregiver. All parties should have a clear understanding of the reasons for the placement and the purposes it serves.

Preparation of the Child

CWLA's *Best Practice Guidelines on Child Maltreatment in Foster Care* (Calhoun, Kaplan, & Williams, 2003) indicate that agencies can help children and youth during the initial transition into foster care by providing them with information about a range of issues:

- the range of feelings such as anger, depression, denial, loss, and confusion that children and youth may experience when placed outside their families;

- the changes and challenges facing children and youth placed outside their homes;

- the roles and expectations of foster parents, agency workers, and birthparents in supporting the placement;

- information about the family they may be placed with, such as lifestyle, description, and pictures;

- the process of case planning and permanency decisionmaking;

- the reasons for their placement, the issues that must be addressed for reunification to occur, and the services and supports that the agency will offer the child and the family to support the reunification process;

- the importance of communicating their feelings and needs to foster parents and agency workers; and

- effective ways to negotiate and resolve conflicts in foster care.

This information should be delivered in the context of an ongoing, supportive relationship with a worker who will be available to support the child through the placement process.

Additional preparation that specifically addresses the prevention of missing-from-care episodes may be necessary, depending on the individual child's history or the worker's assessment of the child's risk:

- For children with a history of running, or who are at risk of running according to the worker's assessment (see Safety and Risk Assessments), the child welfare agency should ensure the availability of education about the short- and long-term risks of running as well as access to information about community-based programs, such as shelter and runaway programs, that provide safety and confidentiality if the child does run.

- Children being transferred between placements may be more likely to go missing just as the transfer is being made. Additional diligence, support, and sensitivity to the needs of the child may be particularly critical at this point.

- For children at risk of family abduction, the worker should provide the child with training on what to do in situations that may put the child at risk, such as unauthorized attempts by parents to pick the child up from school and so forth. Such training must be as nonthreatening as possible, particularly for younger children who are at the greatest risk of family abduction (Hammer et al., 2002). The foster parents should also receive training from the worker so that they can repeat and reinforce learning as needed.

- For all children, the child welfare agency should ensure the availability of age-appropriate education in the prevention of nonfamily member abduction. Ideally, this will be part of a school- or community-based program available to and directed at all children, not targeted specifically to children in out-of-home care. If such a program is not already available, the child welfare agency should work with the local law enforcement agency and schools to develop and initiate one in the community. Barring that, the child welfare agency should collaborate with law enforcement to develop and present a program for youth in care that can be presented as some combination of group training in peer support groups, joint parent-child training in foster parent association groups, and individual informational materials.

Preparation of the Caregiver

For foster parents and staff at group homes and residential facilities, in addition to preservice training that provides grounding in the values, knowledge, and skills necessary to care for all children, the child welfare agency should provide preparation prior to each placement that covers specific information about the individual child, including:

- the child's strengths;
- any academic, social, developmental, behavioral, emotional, or physical challenges the child faces;
- the child's likes and dislikes about living arrangements, foods, sports, recreational activities, animals and pets, religious observances, and so forth;
- any history of running from the birthfamily or previous placements;
- any history of parental abductions or attempted abductions;
- any history of victimization, and the child's emotional and behavioral reactions to maltreatment, that may put the child at increased risk of further victimization or abduction; and

- any increased risk of family or nonfamily abduction the child faces, based on input from current and previous child welfare workers.

Preparation of the Birthfamily

Child welfare agencies should provide preparation and support for families whose children are entering out-of-home care. Agencies should include parents in preplacement decisionmaking and the identification of the child's strengths and needs at the time of placement and also in all subsequent decisionmaking of the service and permanency planning teams.

Birthparents need the same type of preplacement information as agencies provide to children. Misunderstandings and undue anxiety can be avoided if the birthparents are able to understand their children's behavior as they transition into foster care. Birthparents are less likely to feel isolated and alienated from the process when the agency's workers have provided them with information about the foster family and included them in the matching process.

Except when it is not safely possible, agency policy and practice should endorse and facilitate birthparents' communication with and development of relationships with foster parents. This can promote the birthparents' support of the child's placement. Birthparents who feel accepted and respected by foster parents, and who have a firsthand knowledge of the foster parents' concern for their child and competence as caregivers, are more likely to be accepting, if not supportive, of the child's placement in care. This is a special relationship that usually requires facilitation and care to address trust and power issues that may be threatening to either the birthparents or the foster parents. Birthparents who receive adequate preparation for the out-of-home placement of their child may contribute to the prevention of missing episodes by:

- participating in regular visitation with the child;
- encouraging the child to remain in the placement and not run away;
- being available as a support to the child during placement;
- providing the foster family, group home, or residential care staff, or the child welfare worker, with information to complete safety and risk assessments; and

- accepting the child's placement and working with the agency and foster family toward reunification, rather than attempting to remove or keep the child without permission.

Safety and Risk Assessments

The agency should include safety and risk assessments as part of its comprehensive, individualized assessments of the child and the family to determine the appropriate type and level of family foster care or group or residential care. Table 2 shows child factors that agencies should consider pertaining to the prevention of missing-from-care episodes.

Hoff (2002) identified potential indicators of family abduction risk, which are not specific to situations in which the child is in out-of-home care. Indicators are whether the parent has:

- previously abducted the child;
- threatened to abduct the child;
- no strong ties to the child's home state;
- friends or family living out of state or in another country;
- a strong support network;
- no job, is able to work anywhere, or is financially independent—in other words, is not tied to the area for financial reasons;
- engaged in planning activities such as quitting a job, selling a home, terminating a lease, closing a bank account or liquidating other assets, hiding or destroying documents, undergoing plastic surgery, or applying for a passport, birth certificates, or school or medical records;
- a history of marital instability, lack of cooperation with the other parent, or domestic violence or child abuse; or
- a criminal record.

In addition, Hoff (2002) described six personality profiles that may be helpful in predicting which parents may pose a risk of abduction. These are parents who:

- have threatened to abduct or have abducted previously;
- are suspicious or distrustful due to the agency's belief that abuse has occurred and have support for these beliefs;

Table 2. Child Factors Pertaining to Preventing Missing-from-Care Episodes

RISK FACTOR	PROTECTIVE FACTOR
• Previous running from home or placement • Substance abuse • School problems, especially frequent truancy • Involvement with criminal activity • Difficulties with peers, including bullying and harassment • Mental health issues, especially depression, self-harming (e.g, cutting), and suicidal ideation	• Trusting relationship with a caregiver based on mutual respect • Strong connection with at least one adult • Strong relationships with family, friends, peers, and teachers • Strong social and problem-solving skills

- are paranoid delusional;

- are severely sociopathic;

- have strong ties to another country and are ending a mixed-culture marriage; or

- feel alienated from the legal system for reasons such as poverty, membership in a minority group, or previous victimization, and have family and social support in another community.

When assessing the risk of possible family abduction from out-of-home care, the worker should take these profiles into account. Workers should also give special consideration to situations in which:

- someone has made a threat of abduction;

- there have been previous abductions or significant delays in returning child;

- a parent has difficulty separating his or her needs from those of the child; or

- a parent displays hostility toward the agency, caseworker, or foster parent.

Placement Selection and Placement Stability

Running from care is strongly associated with not having a stable placement. The child welfare agency should provide a range of placement options, including kinship care, family foster care, therapeutic family foster care, independent living, and residential care to meet children's individual needs in the most appropriate and least restrictive manner. Caseworkers should select placements that meet children's unique needs to lessen the likelihood of running away. Providing young people with a greater choice of placements and offering them a stable, positive placement experience and a chance to build secure attachments is protective. If placement stability is lacking, youth are less likely to establish a stable pattern of attachments. A trusting relationship with a caregiver based on mutual respect is likely to be the best safeguard for a child (Department of Health, 2002). Placement stability also facilitates the development of strategies to address the underlying difficulties that may have influenced running behavior in the past and has the potential of affecting future behavior.

Children should be placed with kin whenever it is possible to safely do so,* and when relative care is not possible, in the "least restrictive (most family like) setting available" (Adoption Assistance and Child Welfare Act of 1980 [P.L. 96-272], Section 475 [5][A]). Placing children with kin can significantly reduce the likelihood of running away. A search for potential kin placements should begin at the family's initial contact with the child welfare agency through discussions with the birthfamily, the child, and others who know the family to identify family members who can act as supports and, if necessary, as placement options for the child and the birthfamily. Caseworkers should take preferences of children, their parents, and their extended family members into account when multiple kin placements are available.

Because placement with relatives is not possible for all children who enter care, it is essential that child welfare agencies diligently pursue the recruitment of potential foster families that reflect the ethnic and racial diversity of children in the jurisdiction for whom foster homes are needed, which will enable them to select the most appropriate placement for each child coming into care. The child welfare agency should:

- identify the characteristics of the children and youth in need of out-of-home care in their jurisdiction;

- identify the characteristics of families most likely to respond to

---

* The Personal Responsibility and Work Opportunities Reconciliation Act directs that states "shall consider giving preference to an adult relative over a non-related care giver when determining a placement for a child, provided that the relative care giver meets all relevant State child protection standards" (Title IV-E Foster Care and Adoption Assistance State Plan, SEC. 471. [42 U.S.C. 671] [a] [19]).

recruitment efforts, beginning with an understanding of families currently providing foster care services in the jurisdiction; and

- craft and deliver messages designed to be heard by and appeal to potential foster parents in the community.

With a range of placement options from which to choose, agencies should match each child with the family, group home, or residential facility that is best able to meet the child's needs. Factors to consider when making any match are listed in CWLA's Standards of Excellence for Family Foster Care Services (1995). When a child is at increased risk of running away or being abducted by a parent, agencies must consider additional factors in selecting the most appropriate foster family for a given child:

- the family's previous experience with children who have run or been abducted;

- the family's previous success in preventing missing-from-care episodes or dealing with the child in a appropriate manner once the child is returned (see Chapter 6, Return and Resolution); and

- proximity to the child's parents or other family members. Although placement in the same community is generally desirable, when a serious risk of family abduction places the child at risk of harm, a more geographically distant placement may be in the child's better interest. Safety and risk assessments that considers parental factors is the agency's best approach. No assessment, however, can predict the probability of family abduction with 100% certainty.

In addition, caseworkers should match children at increased risk of running away with foster families who have received training in dealing with the behavioral and emotional problems common among such youth, who are committed to continuing to remain a resource for the youth regardless of the occurrence of running episodes, and who are skilled in empathy and the building, sustaining, and repairing of relationships necessary to successfully welcome a youth back from a running episode. Workers should match children at risk of family abduction with foster families who have received training in identifying potential "red flags" and protecting the safety and confidentiality of children, who maintain positive collaborative relationships with the school and other community systems, and who are able to provide a sense of safety and security for the child.

Supporting the Placement

Once the child is placed, the child welfare agency and its staff should support the child, the foster family, and the birthfamily in ways that continue to ensure the child's safety and well-being while working toward permanency. Support includes attention to:

- the child, through worker-child visiting;

- the birthfamily and the child, through parent-child visiting; and

- the foster family, by providing the services and resources required to meet the needs of the family and the child.

Additional supports that can bolster positive development and insulate youth from the risks of running away include: other nurturing relationships, such as mentors, who will remain in the youth's life for a sustained period of time; provision of appropriate medical, psychological, and educational services; and opportunities to participate in normative peer activities (e.g., extracurricular activities, clubs, etc.).

Worker-Child Visitation

A clear correlation exists between regular worker-child visiting and a number of positive outcomes for children in out-of-home care, including preserving children's connections while in care, maintaining children's relationship with parents, and assessing needs and providing services to children and families (U.S. DHHS, n.d.). Visiting provides an opportunity for the child welfare worker and child to develop the type of supportive relationship based on mutual respect that is the single best safeguard against running away. Worker-child visiting should:

- **Occur regularly.** CWLA's *Standards of Excellence for Family Foster Care Services* (1995) recommend monthly visits as a minimum standard, with more frequent visits "if required by the needs of the child or requested by foster parents" (§2.29). Workers, with supervisory input, should schedule more frequent visits if a safety or risk assessment indicates that the child is at increased risk of running away.

- **Include face to face contact with and observation of the child.** There is no substitute for personal contact between the worker and the child.

- **Be meaningful.** Workers should use visiting as a time to listen carefully to what the child has to say about his or her family situation, placement, immediate needs, and long-term goals. Workers should employ listening and relationship-building skills to facilitate the building of trust and respect.

- **Be conducted in an age-, developmentally, and culturally appropriate manner and occur in a relaxed, risk-free environment.** Children are more likely to communicate openly during visits in a home or community setting.

- **Be responsive.** Workers should return phone calls from children promptly, be on time for visits, and be respectful of children's time for school, studying, and other activities. Requests or complaints should result in actions that are responsive to the child's expressed desires or in explanations that provide justification for denial of a request.

- **Be supplemented with additional contacts.** Workers should interview caregivers and other adults and children in the home or at a location of import to the child to obtain a complete picture of the strengths of the child and the caregivers as well as the challenges faced by both in maintaining the stability of the placement.

Parent-Child Visitation

Regular visits with parents, as well as siblings and other kin, protect against missing-from-care episodes by maintaining family relationships for children in care. Children who have access to their families are less likely to run away from care to be with them. They will have less difficulty adjusting to the disruption of family life and will not feel abandoned by their parents. With regular visits, parents are more likely to maintain a feeling of connection to their children and are better able to provide ongoing emotional support. Parents who have contact are more likely to work toward overcoming barriers to reunification. To this end, whenever considered to be safe and appropriate, the service plan should include visits with birthparents at the greatest frequency and longest duration—up to daily visits of several hours—possible given the ability of the child and the birth- and foster families to accommodate them into their schedules. Visits with other kin and especially with siblings should also occur at least weekly, and should take place in the least restrictive setting possible. Determining frequency, length, and setting for visits with birthparents and other family members should take the following factors into consideration:

- the safety of the child;
- the strength and quality of the attachment;
- the child's desire to spend time with parents, siblings, or other kin; and
- the intended role of visits in the service plan and in permanency planning.

Where safety and risk assessments indicate an increased risk of family abduction, parent-child visits should continue to take place. Supervised visitation, in the presence of a third party responsible for observing and ensuring the safety of the child, becomes an important vehicle to maintain connections for both child and parents. Supervised visits are designed to assure that a child can have safe and appropriate contact with an absent parent.

Services and Supports to Foster Families

Placement stability relies on the ability of foster families to deal with the individual needs of the children in their homes as well as the general retention of licensed families who remain with the agency over time and continue to be willing to accept children into their homes. Foster parents are more likely to stay with an agency if:

- workers share information freely, provide ready access to support, and respect and appreciate the parents' contributions to the child welfare team;
- workers validate the import of their relationship with their child and work collaboratively to achieve a mutually agreed-on plan for the child and family;
- a supportive network of caseworkers and other, more experienced foster parents is available for consultation when challenges and crises occur; and
- the agency offers respite on a regular basis.

Foster parents need ongoing inservice training to develop the skills that can enable them to deter children from unauthorized absences and the understanding and competence to follow prescribed agency procedures when children leave care without permission. Failure to report a missing child promptly due to misunderstanding or fear of repercussions may ultimately result in a child being lost in care.

Agencies should also promote and assist in the development of foster parent mentoring relationships and support groups. These support networks can be an invaluable resource to foster parents and kinship caregivers while extending the capacity of the agency to empower foster parents with knowledge and skills.

Services and Supports to Children

Children who receive a full range of services and supports to meet their educational, recreational, and physical and mental health needs while in out-of-home care may be less likely to run away than those who do not. Children and youth are more likely to run if their days have little structure and if their underlying needs are not being satisfactorily addressed. This is especially so in the case of therapeutic services; adolescents who need mental health services and receive adequate therapeutic help are much less likely to run than those who do not (Fasulo, Cross, Mosely, & Leavey, 2002). The caseworker, based on a comprehensive assessment of the child's strengths and needs, and in collaboration with the child, the birthfamily, and the foster family, should develop a service plan that addresses the child's developmental, educational, physical and mental health, recreational, and social needs through both formal service delivery via community providers and informal means, such as school, family, neighborhood, faith-based, and other normative experiences.

Transition Services for Older Youth

All young people in care should receive services provided as part of a comprehensive, long-term plan that includes the activities necessary to prepare for eventual self-sufficiency, as defined in CWLA's Standards of Excellence for Transition, Independent Living, and Self-Sufficiency Services (2005). The engagement of young people in meaningful, individualized plans that address their future needs and connect them with adults who care about them will protect against running episodes.

The caseworker, in collaboration with the child, the birthfamily, and the foster family, should develop a service plan based on a comprehensive assessment of the child's strengths and needs that addresses the child's developmental progress toward independent living. This plan should include, when necessary, the development of basic lifeskills in financial management; educational and employment or vocational competencies; locating and maintaining a safe, stable, affordable place to live; and accessing physical and mental health services. Service plans for young people ages 14 and older should begin to incorporate the development of living skills and knowledge necessary to become independent and interdependent adults. The development of independent lifeskills plans that are responsive to the needs of individual young people and implemented through supportive relationships with caring adults such as foster parents or mentors may dissuade young people for whom the impetus to run is an attraction to the idea of immediate independent living.

In the event a youth does run from care, the knowledge and skills learned in independent living programs may serve to enable him or her to make a safer, more successful transition to independence, even if it is premature and without the continued supervision of the agency.

Services and Supports to Birthfamilies

The agency should provide parents working toward reunification with their children the services they need to support, strengthen, and preserve their family functioning to the fullest extent possible. When service plans are individualized to meet the needs of the family, time limited in accordance with ASFA regulations, and sufficient to enable the child to return safely home, parents are more likely to adhere to the plan and work for reunification and are less likely to attempt to subvert the placement by explicitly or implicitly encouraging children to run from care or by taking their children from care without the permission of the court or agency.

The Role of Information Technology in Prevention

The agency should use regular reports of the location of all children in care, cross-checked with reports of worker-child visiting, to identify potential lost-in-care episodes. Performing such checks on a regular basis enables the agency to identify potential problems swiftly and take action to determine the child's location and status without delay.

On an aggregate level, the collection and analysis of individual, environmental, and systemic factors for all children in care will lead, over time, to a greater ability to identify the risks and protective factors associated with missing-from-care episodes. Agencies can incorporate such factors in and enhance the quality of risk assessments for all children.

Summary

Prevention of missing-from-care episodes is the responsibility of all the individuals who work with the child and his or her family throughout the life of their involvement with the child welfare system. Before placement begins, the agency must adequately prepare the child, the caregiver, and the child's family. Family-centered practice and individualized strengths-based assessment and planning form the basis of this preparation of all parties. Preparation should include safety and risk assessmentd that take into account risk factors that may increase the likelihood of running or family abduction, as well as protective factors that indicate the child will be well supported in the foster family.

Optimal prevention begins with careful selection of a foster family, group, or residential placement that meets the individual needs of the child in the least restrictive environment possible and provides the child with a trusting relationship with a caregiver based on mutual respect. Placement with a relative is generally the most desirable placement setting; if that is not possible, the caseworker should try to match the child's needs with a foster family, group, or residential facility best suited to meet those needs.

Once the child is in care, the agency must support the placement with worker-child visits, parent-child visits, and services and supports for the child, the parent, and the foster family. Older adolescents should receive appropriate transition services to help them prepare for the future, regardless of their permanency plan. Agencies can use their management informatin systems to identify potentially missing children quickly as well as to build a body of knowledge that will lead to improved understanding of the risk factors associated with missing-from-care episodes.

CHAPTER 5

Responding to Children Missing from Care

Once a child has gone missing from out-of-home care, the child welfare agency must respond swiftly and decisively and do everything in its power to locate the missing child and return him or her to a safe environment. It is essential that the agency work collaboratively with the law enforcement agency to produce the quickest and best outcome possible for each missing child.

Before a child goes missing from out-of-home care, the agency should have a written plan in place for all areas of response, beginning with a procedure for making appropriate notifications. Child welfare agencies should write such procedures into any MOUs with the law enforcement agency. This chapter makes recommendations for procedures that should be followed in responding to a missing child episode as well as detailed in MOUs.

Single Point of Contact

The child welfare agency should designate a single point of contact, with 24-hour, 7-day a week availability, for the receipt and notification of all missing episodes. The individual responsible for this point of contact should receive special training in all procedures to be followed regarding each type of missing episode. The agency should ensure that all potential reporters are familiar with reporting procedures and with how to access the designated point of contact. People responsible for manning the single point of contact should have immediate access to:

- the agency administrator, the agency's general counsel, and the director of public relations or public affairs;
- contact information for all caseworkers, foster parents, and children in care;
- a single point of contact with the local law enforcement agency;
- all individual case records; and

- management information reports detailing the location of all children in care in the jurisdiction.

Notifications

MOUs between the child welfare and law enforcement agencies should detail specific actions to be taken by each agency regarding notifications, including points of contact at each agency and a time line of actions.

Taking the Initial Report

The first report that a child is missing from care will generally come from the child's caregiver or will be reported directly to the child welfare agency (see Figure 1). Caregivers and other potential reporters should be familiar with and have access to written copies of procedures for making appropriate notifications.

Foster Parent. A foster parent will frequently be the first person to become aware of a missing child, whether the child has run away or been abducted. Unless agency policy dictates otherwise, foster parents should be instructed to report a child as a runaway or potential runaway if the child is missing for 12 hours or overnight, or earlier if any of the circumstances or child characteristics described in the definition of runaway (see Chapter 1) are present, or if the foster parent for any other reason believes the child has run away.

The foster parent should notify the first of these individuals he or she can reach, in this order: (a) the child's social worker, (b) the worker's supervisor, (c) the designated point of contact in the child welfare agency, or (d) the local law enforcement agency. Agency protocol should specify both the sequence of contacts and the individuals to be contacted. In cases in which the child is missing in the course of the commission of a crime, such as if the child is abducted from the foster parent's custody, or may be in immediate danger, the first contact should be the law enforcement agency; the foster parent should then also contact the child's social worker, the worker's supervisor, or the designated point of contact in the child welfare agency, whoever he or she can reach first.

Group Home or Residential Care Staff. Group homes and residential facilities should ensure that a single individual or office is responsible for receiving all reports of missing children, 24 hours a day, 7 days a week. When a child is missing from a group or residential care facility, the staff member

Figure 1. Responding to Children Missing-from-Care Episodes

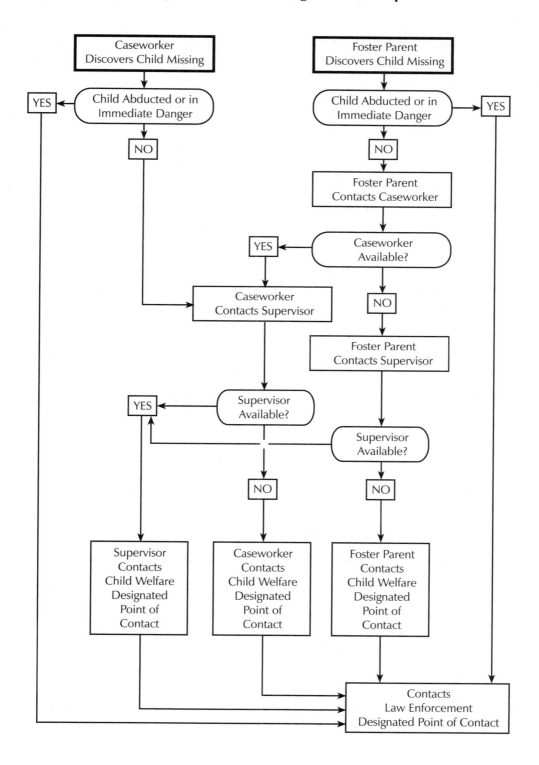

should report immediately to a designated person or office at the facility, who should then follow the same procedures as those expected of a foster parent.

Caseworker or Other Child Welfare Agency Staff. The child's caseworker or other agency staff may be the first to be aware of a child's status as missing or possibly missing from care. If the worker suspects that a child may be missing (i.e., the child fails to appear at an appointment or is not present at an expected location, such as at school or a medical examination), the caseworker should first call the foster parent. If the foster parent does not know the child's whereabouts, the caseworker and foster parent together should attempt to locate the child by checking with the child's friends, neighbors, and relatives. If they are unable to determine the location of the child in fairly short order, and no longer than 12 hours or overnight, the caseworker should notify his or her supervisor and the designated agency point of contact. If the caseworker is unable to reach either of those individuals, or has knowledge that the child is missing in connection with the commission of a crime or may be in immediate danger, he or she should contact the law enforcement agency.

The child welfare agency staff member who receives the initial report, whether he or she is the worker, supervisor, or designated point of contact, should ascertain as much of the following information as possible from the reporter:

- the child's name;
- the child's age;
- any physical or psychological conditions, such as developmental delays, that might affect the ability of the child to respond to dangers in the environment;
- a physical description, including clothes the child was wearing when last seen;
- medications or a history of suspected substance abuse;
- the type of missing episode (runaway, family abduction, nonfamily abduction);
- the immediate circumstances of the disappearance;
- the names and addresses of the foster parents, birthparents, relatives, former foster parents, and friends;

- locations and activities the child is known to frequent;
- any suspected destinations; and
- any prior disappearances and outcomes.

The agency staff member should then obtain the child's case file to ascertain any of the above information not known by the reporter and to gather a photograph taken in the last six months if the child is younger than 6, or the last 12 months if the child is older and a copy of the most recent court order granting legal custody of the child.

All reports of missing children, whether received by the caseworker, supervisor, or other agency staff, should be provided to the agency point of contact, who will then notify the law enforcement agency.

Notification of the Law Enforcement Agency

Following the procedures described here, the child welfare agency or foster parent should notify the law enforcement agency in every case of a child missing from care. Whenever feasible, the contact should be between designated single points of contact in each of the two agencies. Contact should be first by telephone, followed by written notification. If the law enforcement agency becomes aware of a missing-from-care episode before the child welfare agency, it should notify the child welfare agency through the designated single point of contact.

When a child is missing, law enforcement personnel must have access to the information about the child, the child's placement, and the child's family that will enable them to conduct an investigation; the goal of this investigation is the swift, safe return of the child. MOUs should specify the information to be shared with law enforcement. For information not covered by MOUs, consultation with the agency administrator and agency counsel is advised, and the child welfare agency should authorize its representative (the single point of contact) to release this information once approval has been received. Sample forms for the collection of information are provided in Appendices B, C, and D. MOUs should include any specific format designated by the agencies involved. Generally, the law enforcement agency should be given the following information about the child at the first notification:

- full name;
- aliases and nicknames, if any;
- age and date of birth;

- Social Security number;

- drivers' license number, if applicable;

- a comprehensive physical description including height, weight, hair color, eye color, skin color, and information such as presence of braces, contact lenses, dentures, gold or silver teeth, impairment (hearing, vision, speech), moles, scars, body piercings, or tattoos;

- any physical or psychological conditions, such as developmental delays, that might affect the ability of the child to respond to dangers in the environment;

- other factors of endangerment, such as young age, hazardous location, need for medical attention, or disability;

- medications or history of suspected substance abuse;

- photograph taken within the last 6 months if the child is younger than 6, or last 12 months if the child is older;

- a copy of the most recent court order granting legal custody of the child and other relevant facts about child's custody status;

- type of missing episode (runaway, family abduction, nonfamily abduction, "lost" in care);

- where, when, and with whom the child was last seen;

- clothing worn, including eyeglasses, hat, book bag, shoes, and so forth;

- possible method of travel, such as vehicle, bicycle, public transportation, or on foot;

- names and addresses of foster parents, birthparents, relatives, former foster parents, and friends;

- locations and activities the child is known to frequent;

- any suspected destinations; and

- any prior disappearances and outcomes.

In addition to the information provided at the initial notification of law enforcement, the child welfare agency should be prepared to provide law enforcement with access to caseworkers who can give additional information that may be relevant to locating the child, which may include the child's developmental or behavioral history and family dynamics and history.

Notification of the Birthfamily

The child's birthfamily should be notified immediately and, whenever feasible, in person, of any missing-from-care episode. Because it is possible that a runaway child will return to the birthfamily, as well as the potential occurrence of family abduction, the notification should be made by child welfare and law enforcement agencies together, in the context of the initial investigatory interview (see below).

Notification of the Court

The agency should file a motion with the court in accordance with the time frame established by agency policy, optimally within two working days of the initial report of the child's status as missing. The motion should include efforts being made to locate the child.

Safety and Risk Assessments

The caseworker should assess and document the relative safety and risk for each child who goes missing from out-of-home care. Factors to be taken into account in considering the relative risk of harm to any individual child include:

- age;
- developmental status;
- physical or mental disability;
- need for medication;
- vulnerability to maltreatment or exploitation, based on history of abuse and neglect;
- history of running or missing episodes;
- absence inconsistent with established pattern of behavior; and
- circumstances of the child's disappearance.

The caseworker's assessment of the child's level of risk should be shared with law enforcement personnel. For law enforcement agencies, NCMEC (2000, p. 29) identifies a list of "unusual circumstances" that heighten risk and prompt an immediate and full-scale response (see Appendix C).

The Investigation

The law enforcement agency should take the lead on any missing child investigation. The child welfare agency has the following responsibilities in its partnership with law enforcement:

- make contacts and conduct inquiries as requested by law enforcement personnel,

- provide information as requested by the law enforcement agency through the designated agency contacts,

- keep law enforcement updated with any new or changed information, and

- request status reports at regular intervals.

Initial Interviews

Initial interviews, including notification of missing status, with foster parents, group home or residential care staff, and birthparents should take place in face-to-face-meetings at which law enforcement and child welfare personnel are present. A multidisciplinary approach both reassures the adults who are concerned about the safety of the child and ensures that all information is shared fully and directly with both agencies.

Both agencies have the safety of the child as their first concern. Each agency has its own functions in the interview process and brings an essential area of expertise to the interview. The child welfare agency representative should:

- present information about the child's status to the birthparents, foster parents, or group home or residential care staff;

- advise interviewees of their right to give informed consent, if applicable; and

- assist interviewees in determining the limits of confidentiality in releasing information about the child or the child's family.

The law enforcement agency should assume the lead role in the investigative interview. The caseworker should expect to be interviewed by law enforcement and be prepared to answer questions based on his or her own relationship with the missing child.

Ongoing Investigation

Throughout the time the child is missing, the child welfare and law enforcement agencies should maintain a schedule of contacts. Depending on the type of missing-from-care episode and the terms of any MOU, this may include regularly scheduled multidisciplinary meetings, phone or e-mail updates, and sharing of MIS or other computerized reports.

Each agency should update the other through a mutually agreed-on procedure when they receive new or updated information concerning the child. The child welfare agency should share any changes in contact information for the child's birthfamily, friends, relatives, and foster family with the law enforcement agency.

Efforts to solicit information about the child's location should be made and documented regularly as described in the interagency MOU. Caseworkers may be responsible for contacting family members, friends, and other individuals who may have knowledge of the child's whereabouts in some cases, such as runaways and children "lost" in care.

When the Child Turns 18

The goal for a youth is to leave care with an individualized transition plan for moving toward interdependence. Young people who go missing in the absence of such a plan, regardless of their age, are unlikely to have achieved a sense of permanency before leaving care. Youth who leave care without the skills and a plan for independence experience problems that make transitioning into adult life an enormous challenge. A critical element of the plan should be to identify adults with whom the youth can establish or strengthen lifelong connections.

While in care, it is extremely important for youth to define family connections for themselves. Family connections are people a young person has or has had a supportive relationship with, such as relatives, former foster parents, group home staff, school personnel, or other professionals. Transitional support services to young people should maintain a strong focus on building supportive relationships and establishing support systems within the community (CWLA, 2005).

When a child turns 18 while in missing status, state statute or agency regulations or policy should dictate whether the caseworker may close the child welfare case. Whether the case is closed or remains open, the case record and MIS should maintain a record of the child as being missing. The child welfare agency should inform the law enforcement agency if the child welfare case is closed.

If the missing person is located after the child welfare case is closed, the law enforcement agency should notify the child welfare agency, which can then update its MIS. Notification of others, including the birthfamily, siblings, other relatives, or foster parents may be made, depending on the facts of the individual case and the wishes of the formerly missing person. If the located child is deceased, all notifications should be made.

Interjurisdictional Issues

When the child is in placement outside of the home jurisdiction, the child welfare agency should immediately notify the agency from which the child came. That agency should then enter the status of the child as missing into its own MIS or case record and be prepared to cooperate with law enforcement in the investigation of the case.

The child welfare agency of the child's home jurisdiction may have information useful to locating the child, including but not limited to contact information for local family members and friends, records of past missing-from-care episodes, and birthfamily dynamics and history. The local law enforcement agency may also have information such as criminal records of the child or a possible abductor or records of past missing-from-care investigations. If the child has run away or been abducted by a family member, the destination may be to the originating jurisdiction.

Both child welfare and law enforcement agencies in the jurisdiction in which the child goes missing should contact their counterparts in the child's home jurisdiction and report the child's status as missing from out-of-home care. It is essential that both agencies share information and updates with their counterparts in other jurisdictions.

Juvenile Justice Involvement

Children and youth who run away from out-of-home care may come in contact with the juvenile justice system as a result of criminal activity or may be picked up for truancy or vagrancy. When children in foster care are arrested for delinquent acts, they are more likely than other children to be sent to juvenile detention to await their trials, rather than back home. Not having a person to release a child to is one reason court officials may detain juveniles. Foster youth who are detained for several consecutive days could lose their foster care placements (Ross, 2001).

Frontline workers are not always aware of a youth's involvement in other systems. A youth may be identified as missing from care when in fact he or she is in the juvenile justice system. Some law enforcement officers may not ask if the youth is in foster care. It is critical for system collaboration that caseworkers be well informed and provide relevant information to the court (Ross, 2001). MOUs between child welfare and law enforcement agencies should address how the law enforcement search for the missing child is coordinated with the juvenile justice and the child welfare systems.

The Role of Information Technology in Investigation and Response

Management Information Systems (MIS)

The child welfare agency's MIS should contain data elements that enable the agency to enter the following information:

- missing status,
- date missing status was reported,
- last verified caseworker contact with the child,
- date the agency notified law enforcement, and
- date agency notified court.

Ideally, the child welfare agency's system should interface automatically with that of the law enforcement agency, which should in turn notify the NCIC Missing Person File. If the system does not, MOUs should address procedures for manual interface so that the systems contain consistent, up-to-date information.

Identification of Children "Lost" in Care

Agencies should generate weekly MIS reports that cross-check the location of all children against reports of visits by caseworkers and identify children whose whereabouts are in question or unknown. Caseworkers should verify the location of all children identified this way immediately with personal contact visits, and supervisors should review all reports of visits. Children not located should be considered missing and treated as such.

Websites

Making information available on websites about children who are missing has proven to be an effective means of locating them. The child welfare agency may choose to post pictures of missing children on an Internet website accessible to the general public. The urgent need to locate and ensure the safety of children supersedes concerns about confidentiality, including disclosing the identity of children in out-of-home care. Information posted on a website may include the child's photograph, name, age, physical description, and location where he or she was last seen.

Internet listing should be avoided in cases in which publication of the child's identity, photograph, or description may place him or her at greater risk. An example of such circumstances would be potential targeting of a runaway child by a family member or other party.

Supporting Caregivers, Birthparents, and Other Children in Care

When a child goes missing from care, the families and others who care about the child will be under stress and may be traumatized by the circumstances of the episode, particularly if abduction is involved. The caseworker should update birthparents, foster parents, and siblings of the missing child regularly about the status of the investigation, even if no new information has been discovered. It is essential to assure families and siblings that the child welfare and law enforcement agencies are doing everything possible to locate the missing child.

The caseworker should provide extra supports to birthparents, siblings, and foster parents during the missing-from-care episode, including extending access to him- or herself or another agency representative for phone calls and counseling. Birthparents may be particularly concerned about the safety of any of their other children who are in out-of-home care. The caseworker should make every effort to assure the parent about the safety of their children and provide opportunities for the parent and children to be in frequent contact, including visits, telephone calls, and e-mails. This will reassure the children, who are likely to be concerned about the safety of their sibling.

The distress of foster parents related to the episode should not be forgotten or downplayed. The caseworker should provide those foster parents who have other children in their home with respite care to relieve stress and provide an opportunity for breaks from caregiving.

If the missing child was abducted, siblings of the child and other children in the foster home should be escorted to and from school and other activities. If the foster parents are unable to do so, the caseworker should assist them in finding people who can perform this task.

Supporting Agency Staff

Caseworkers and other agency staff may also be affected by missing-from-care episodes, and the agency should take care to ensure that supervisors and managers are trained in understanding the ways such episodes contribute to stress. Training should focus on the identification and management of stress and trauma in individual staff as well as the potential adverse effects on performance of the individual and the workforce as a whole.

Caseworkers and other staff who work with the missing child, the child's family, or the foster family should receive support through frequent contact with supervisors and opportunities to discuss events and their reactions to them. Managers should share information about the investigation with staff who are involved with the child's case. In the case of abduction where the child is in danger, or if the child is harmed or killed while missing, the episode is elevated to the status of a critical incident, and the agency should support staff through critical incident stress debriefing.

Critical Incident Stress Debriefing

Events that are traumatic to people, including the serious harm to or death of children in one's care, are considered critical incidents. People exposed to one or more critical incidents are subject to critical incident stress (Mitchell, 1983). The International Critical Incident Stress Foundation (n.d.) lists a range of physical, cognitive, emotional, and behavioral symptoms that have the potential to interfere with one's ability to perform effectively both on and off the job. Without appropriate action following a critical incident, serious and long-term consequences may result.

Child welfare agencies should develop a plan and identify resources and protocols for debriefing critical incidents. Responses may include debriefing by trained peer support staff, external crisis counselors, or employee assistance program counselors; trauma support groups that meet on a regular basis; and peer-to-peer support on a unit level (Friedman, 2002).

Summary

The child welfare agency should be prepared to respond to missing-from-care episodes by having in place an agency plan and MOU with the local law enforcement agency. The plan should provide procedures for identifying a contact person in each agency; notifying appropriate personnel at both agencies, the birthparents, and the court; conducting safety and risk assessments for the missing child; and conducting the initial investigatory interviews.

The conduct of the ongoing investigation is under the purview of the law enforcement agency, but the child welfare agency should continue to solicit information from contacts and keep track of the progress of the case on a regular basis. It should employ information technology, including MIS and Internet listings of missing children, to the fullest extent possible.

Care should be taken to support the birthparents, siblings, and foster parents of children who go missing throughout the missing episode, as well as to attend to the stress experienced by child welfare staff, particularly in critical incidents.

CHAPTER 6

Return and Resolution

The location and return of children missing from care should never be the conclusion of the episode, but rather the beginning of a process designed to:

- attend to the immediate needs of the child, the birthfamily, and the foster family;

- reassess the child's safety, permanence, and well-being;

- reassess the placement, treatment, and permanency plans and make changes as appropriate;

- give feedback to the foster family and the caseworker about strengths as well as challenges and issues that might improve their work with children, and provide training or support as appropriate to help them make necessary improvements; and

- provide information to the child welfare agency about systemic issues that it should use in a continuous quality improvement process to address the problem of children missing from care. Such information and data will add to the body of knowledge about the issue.

Return of the Child

After the child is located, the first task is to return him or her to a safe site. The responsibility and procedure for doing so may depend on the type of missing-from-care episode that occurred as well as the circumstances and the location at which the child is found.

Abducted Child is Located by Law Enforcement Agency

If the child has been abducted and is then located by the law enforcement agency, MOUs between the two agencies should spell out procedures for return to the physical custody of the child welfare agency. A complete agency plan will include a multidisciplinary recovery and reunification team that includes law enforcement and child welfare personnel, mental and physical health professionals, and a victim-witness advocate, all specially trained in the recovery and return of missing children. Turman's (1995) *Recovery and Reunification of Missing Children: A Team Approach* provides guidelines for developing, implementing, and using such teams. In general, the law enforcement agency will take the lead in the return of abducted children. The child welfare agency should be prepared to take physical custody of the child at the location specified by the law enforcement agency, which may be the location at which the child was found, a medical facility, or the law enforcement agency.

Runaway Child is Located by Law Enforcement Agency

Law enforcement procedures on location of a runaway child may vary depending on the circumstances and the child's condition at the time. MOUs between law enforcement and child welfare agencies should detail issues to be considered in determining the procedure to be followed, which may include the child's age, the child's physical and mental condition, people with whom the child was living, victimization or exploitation suffered by the child, and any criminal activity on the part of the child.

In most cases in which a young person has run away and is then safely located, the law enforcement agency will notify the child welfare agency of the child's location. A representative of the child welfare agency should go to the location and take physical custody of the child. The person representing the agency should be someone known to the child and with whom the child has a positive relationship.

Runaway Child is Located by Someone Other Than Law Enforcement

When a child is located, or the child's location is reported to the child welfare agency or caregiver, the child welfare and law enforcement agencies should respond jointly to ensure the safety of the child and facilitate the return of the child to the custody of the child welfare agency.

Runaway Child Returns Voluntarily

When a runaway child returns to the caregiver or the agency on his or her own, the caseworker should notify the law enforcement agency and make an initial contact immediately to ensure the safety of the child. The foster parent or staff at a group home or residential care facility is responsible for immediately notifying the child welfare agency if a child returns voluntarily to the placement.

In all of these situations, a series of activities and interventions should occur (see below) that promote understanding of the missing-from-care episode, inform placement decisions, and determine the need for immediate and long-term services and supports for the child, foster family, and birthfamily.

Notifications

MOUs between the child welfare and law enforcement agencies should detail specific actions each agency should take regarding notifications, including points of contact at each agency and a time line of actions. The caseworker and/or other assigned agency personnel should immediately notify the following people with information about the child's return, condition, and, unless safety is an issue, current location: the birthparents, foster parents, siblings, guardian ad litem or court-appointed special advocate, juvenile court, and law enforcement personnel (in the event that they are unaware of the child's return).

The caseworker should immediately update the child welfare agency's MIS and the child's case file with the child's status. Any information about the child posted on the Internet should be removed immediately. The law enforcement agency should update the NCIC system.

Placement

The child should be returned to his or her last placement following the completion of a comprehensive debriefing interview unless:

- no bed is available for the child,
- the child refuses to return to the placement or states that he or she will run away again immediately,
- the worker has reason to believe the child will be in danger of maltreatment,
- the worker has reason to believe the child will be in danger of abduction, or
- the child's physical or mental condition requires treatment in a hospital or mental health facility.

If the child cannot return to his or her previous placement for one or more of these reasons, the caseworker should determine which placement alternatives is most appropriate for the child. Placement alternatives might include: placement in another family foster home, an emergency or shelter placement, a group home or residential placement, or placement in a hospital or mental health facility. When age- and developmentally appropriate, the child should participate in the decision of what should be clearly represented as a temporary placement until the complete placement planning team meets to review the placement decision.

The worker should inform the child and foster parents or facility staff that a debriefing interview will be conducted within 24 hours and that the child may be moved based on the content of that interview. Once the debriefing interview has been completed (see below), the child's placement may be changed based on changes in the permanency plan, input of the youth, changes in the treatment plan, or input of the foster parent.

Changes in the Permanency Plan

As a result of the interview and subsequent work with the child and the family, the team may revise the child's permanency plan, and a change of placement may be required. Options may include reconsideration of reunification with the birthfamily or permanence with an adoptive family, legal guardian, or in another planned, permanent living arrangement.

Input of the Youth

It is critical that young people themselves are meaningfully and actively involved in the process of making decisions that affect their lives. The issue of permanency, which includes understanding what it means to the young person as well as developing a plan to achieve it, presents an opportunity to actively engage young people in planning for their futures.

Situations that may lead to a change in placement include the following:

- Some young people run from out-of-home care to the home of a relative, including a birthparent, older sibling, or extended family member or other trusted adult. Even though the permanency plan does not change, a change of placement may provide a more stable situation, may enable the youth to maintain connections with family, and may contribute positively to the youth's well-being while in care.

- The youth may express a strong desire to change placements due to a difficult relationship with the current caregiver. The youth may not feel that the caregiver is responsive to his or her needs, may not feel connected to the caregiver, or may desire more autonomy and the opportunity to work on developing skills needed for life after care. In such cases, the youth and caregiver should receive support in this decisionmaking.

- The youth may wish to move to an independent living situation in anticipation of aging out of care. The agency may respect such wishes when it is a developmentally appropriate option for the young person and the agency is able to provide services to support the youth in such a living arrangement. Such an arrangement should in no way be considered a permanent plan for the young person. The child welfare system must strive to help youth in foster care achieve permanency while ensuring that they are learning the skills they need to function as adults.

Changes in the Treatment Plan

The debriefing interview may lead to a determination to provide new or different services and supports to meet the child's developmental, educational, behavioral, and physical or mental health needs, or to step up or down the child's level of care. This may include the need to provide intensive treatment to deal with any trauma the child may have suffered during the missing-from-care episode.

Input of the Foster Parent

The foster parent may ask that the child be moved, either as a direct result of the episode or for other reasons. If the young person expresses a desire to remain with the foster parent, the caseworker should make every effort to work with the foster family and provide additional training and supports if it will be possible to maintain the placement with those services.

In any case in which a placement change will occur, the child and the new foster parent should be prepared in the same way as for an initial placement (see Chapter 4, Prevention).

The Debriefing Interview

Every child who is missing from care should receive an age- and developmentally appropriate debriefing interview within 24 hours of his or her return. When the returned child has been abducted or has been criminally victimized while missing, procedures regarding the conduct of the interview should be covered in the MOU to reduce the number of interviews and lessen the trauma of asking the child to repeat the same information multiple times.

The Interviewer

If the child was abducted or was victimized during a runaway episode, the interview should be conducted by a mental health professional who is a member of the interdisciplinary recovery team. In this instance, the law enforcement agency will be seeking information to help in the criminal investigation, whereas the child welfare agency will want to assess the physical and emotional status of the child.

In other types of episodes, the interview should be conducted by a caseworker or an independent third party selected or approved by the child (e.g., counselor from runaway shelter). The interviewer should be a trusted adult identified as such by the child. The child must feel that the interviewer is nonjudgmental and will maintain confidentiality. Any person who might conduct debriefing interviews should have a combination of education, experience, and training that includes the following competencies:

- knowledge about developmental issues, trauma and attachment, why children run, risks associated with running, placement and permanency options, and the value of the youth's voice in placement and permanency decisions; and

- skill in developmentally appropriate interviewing techniques, establishing rapport, and communicating empathy.

Content of the Interview

The initial debriefing interview, as well as follow-up discussions that may be necessary, should explore the following subjects:

- reasons the child went missing;

- what happened during the episode;

- what supports or services the child needs to cope with those events;

- what the agency, the foster family, the birthfamily, and the child can do to prevent another episode;

- what supports or services the child needs to resolve the issues that led to the episode; and

- alternative options for the child should he or she feel the need to leave care without permission again.

A sample interview guide for such a debriefing interview appears in Appendix D.

After the Interview

The debriefing interview is not the completion of the missing-from-care episode; rather, it is only one step in a continuous process of improving the quality of care for both the individual child and for all children in the care of the agency. Several additional steps should follow the interview.

Safety and Risk Assessments

The caseworker should review and update the safety and risk assessment process described in Chapter 4 and incorporate these assessments into the service, placement, and permanency planning processes described here.

Placement Determination

The caseworker should meet with the service planning team, including the child when developmentally appropriate, the foster family, the birthfamily, and other concerned adults, to review and revise the placement determination. In addition to factors discussed in Chapter 4, the worker should consider issues raised as a result of the episode or during the debriefing interview in determining the most appropriate placement for the child. For some older youth, consideration may be given to a supported independent living setting.

Service Planning and Delivery

The caseworker should meet with the service planning team, including the child when developmentally appropriate, the foster family, the birthfamily, and other concerned adults, to review and revise the service plan. The worker should incorporate services and supports, including health services, to address issues that led to the missing episode and resolve any trauma suffered during the episode into the plan. The revised plan may include a change in placement and may incorporate an independent living skills component.

Permanency Planning

The caseworker should meet with the permanency planning team, including the child, foster family, birthfamily, relatives, and other concerned adults, to review the permanency goal and revise it when necessary and appropriate.

Ongoing Support

The caseworker should increase the frequency of monitoring of the child's well-being, including worker-child and worker-foster parent visiting and phone calls. The caseworker should seek to ensure that the child has a relationship with at least one caring, trusted adult who is concerned about the child. That person may be the foster parent, a relative, a mentor, or another adult, such as a teacher or former caregiver, who can convey to the child a sense of concern for his or her well-being.

Contingency Planning

The caseworker should assist the child in making contingency plans for situations that might lead to a recurrence of the missing-from-care episode, including steps that might be taken instead of leaving care and the location of a safe place to go in the event the child feels the need to leave the placement.

Feedback to the Caseworker

The supervisor should conduct a teaching interview with the caseworker in which they review the episode from beginning to end. The purpose of this interview is to provide constructive feedback to the caseworker on his or her strengths as well as weaknesses in the handling of the case and the episode. It is also to develop an improvement plan, if warranted, that will enable the worker to increase his or her effectiveness in working with children, youth, and families.

Feedback to the Foster Family

Following the teaching interview with his or her supervisor, the caseworker should conduct a teaching interview with the foster family, whether the child has returned to that placement or not. This interview should mirror that conducted by the supervisor. The purpose is to provide constructive feedback to the foster parents on their strengths as well as weaknesses in the handling of the child and the episode and develop an improvement plan, if warranted, that will enable the foster parents to increase their effectiveness in working with children, youth, and families.

Record Keeping

The worker should update the agency's records, including the MIS and the child's individual case record, to reflect information about the episode, as discussed in Chapter 2.

Summary

The child welfare agency should consider the safe return of a child who has been missing from out-of-home care as one step in a continuous process of assessing and ensuring the safety, permanence, and well-being of the child. The safe physical return of the child should be covered by an MOU between the child welfare and law enforcement agencies, and all interested parties should be notified as soon as possible.

Once the child is physically in the custody of the agency and in a safe placement, and based on the type of missing episode, the appropriate team member should conduct a debriefing interview to determine why the child went missing, what happened during the episode, what needs to be done in response to what happened, and what needs to be done to prevent further episodes. The agency should then undertake a series of activities to ensure that the child's placement, services, and permanency planning goals are still appropriate; update them when necessary; and provide needed supports to help the child, the foster family, and the birthfamily deal with the missing-from-care episode and any attending trauma.

Child Welfare and Law Enforcement Agencies Jointly Prepared Procedures

Suggested Activities

- Share contact lists of child welfare supervisors and law enforcement investigators among agencies.

- Share changes in internal processes, policies, and staff members.

- Conduct joint case staffings.

- Create an oversight committee to monitor adherence to policy, strengthen interprofessional processes and practices, and address challenges to successful response and intervention.

- Coordinate joint reporting and data sharing.

- Conduct joint training on policies and procedures, scenario-based training exercises, investigative processes, available technologies, interviewing techniques, and report writing and other documentation procedures.

- Prepare a protocol and train those people at both agencies who receive and respond to telephone calls regarding missing children.

- Define consistent requirements between the child welfare agency intake report and the law enforcement missing persons report.

- Develop a joint initial investigation protocol.

- Enact jointly developed intervention processes.

- Develop an exchange program in which regular duty law enforcement personnel and child welfare staff spend a day working with their counterparts.

- Develop a joint process and forms for interviewing each child who has returned from a missing-from-care episode.

- Develop mutually agreed-on forms for collecting contact information, recording child and family data at intake, reporting a missing child, tracking leads, taking tips, and recording information.

- Create a public information plan to prepare for press coverage in high-profile cases.

Memorandums of Understanding (MOUs) Among Child Welfare and Law Enforcement Agencies: Suggested Elements

- Statement of purpose

- Discussion of joint and respective missions and organizational responsibilities.

- Roles and responsibilities of different professionals.

- Definitions and types of missing-from-care episodes covered.

- Procedures for handling each type of episode, including investigative techniques.

- Procedure for joint response to reports of missing children.

- Establishment of points of contact between agencies and with birthfamilies, foster parents or other caregivers, media, and other community service providers.

- Information to be shared and procedures for sharing information about the child, the family, and the investigation.

- Procedures for return of children once they are located.

- Procedures for debriefing children and families.

- Provisions for joint or cross-training.

- Provisions for multidisciplinary consultation, which will establish the framework for the future addition of other parties to the protocol.

- Criteria and procedures for working with other agencies.

- Concrete tips for handling special issues (e.g., procedures for handling cases not covered by protocol).

- Methods of oversight and evaluation and renewal of agreement.

- Relevant appendices, such as selected portions of statues, regulations, and annotated code, and so forth.

Unusual Circumstances That Prompt an Immediate and Full-Scale Response

- The missing child is 13 years of age or younger.

- The missing child is believed to be out of the zone of safety for his or her age and developmental stage.

- The missing child is mentally incapacitated.

- The missing child is drug dependent, including prescribed medication or illegal substances, and the dependency is potentially life threatening.

- The missing child was absent for more than 24 hours before being reported to the police.

- Based on available information, it is determined that the missing child is in a life-threatening situation.

- Based on available information, it is believed that the missing child is in the company of adults who could endanger his or her welfare.

- The absence is inconsistent with his or her established patterns of behavior, and the deviation cannot be readily explained.

- Other circumstances are involved in the disappearance that would cause a reasonable person to conclude that the child should be considered at risk.

Sample Tools

1. **Kentucky Abducted and Runaway Kids System (ARKS) Information Sheet**

2. **New York State Division of Criminal Justice Services Missing and Exploited Children Clearinghouse: Runaway Checklist**

3. **New York State Division of Criminal Justice Services Missing and Exploited Children Clearinghouse: Family Abduction Checklist**

4. **State of Illinois Department of Children and Family Services: Missing Child De-Briefing Form**

Kentucky Abducted and Runaway Kids System (ARKS) Information Sheet

Date: _____

Child's Name: _____ (as listed on CWS/CMS*)

Child's Date of Birth: _____ Court #: _____ Warrant #: _____

Date of Runaway Event: _____ Date Child Returned: _____

Placement Type at Time of Running Away: (check one category)

❑ Foster Home Foster Family Agency Foster Home   ❑ Group Home
❑ Relative Caregiver/Nonrelative Extended Family Member   ❑ Home of Parent
❑ Nonrelative Legal Guardian
❑ Other (please specify): _____

Reasons/Circumstances for Running Away: (check one main category)

❑ Unknown at this time ❑ Pattern/History of running away ❑ Wish to return home
❑ Left with friends   ❑ Refusal to obey rules   ❑ Avoid (re)placement
❑ Acting-out behavior(s) ❑ Age 18 (or older) & refusing services or detention
❑ Other (please specify): _____

Current Efforts to Locate Child

Party Contacted	Date Contacted	Results
❑ Law enforcement		
❑ Parents/Legal Guardian(s)		
❑ Relatives/Siblings/Nonrelative extended family members		
❑ Former Out-of-Home Caregiver(s)		
❑ Child's Friends		
❑ Former CSWs [Case-Carrying Children's Social Worker		
❑ Child's Former and/or Current School		
❑ Clearances (Single Index, CWS/CMS, JAI)		
❑ Other:		

Other Actions Taken

❑ Notified Child's Attorney   Date_____
❑ Notified Parent(s)/Legal Guardian   Date_____
❑ Protective Custody Warrant Requested/Issued   Date_____
❑ Secured Child's Belongings   Date_____
   Location of belongings _____

CSW's Name: _____ Tel. # _____ File # _____
SCSW's** Name: _____ Tel. # _____

_____

* Child Welfare Services/Case Management System
** Supervisor of Case-Carrying Children's Social Worker

New York State Division of Criminal Justice Services Missing and Exploited Children Clearinghouse: Runaway Checklist*

Reporting Person Information

Date: _____   ❑ Male   ❑ Female

Name: Last _____ First _____ MI _____

Street Address: _____

City/State/ZIP: _____

Relationship to Child: _____

Telephone #: (Home/Work)
(_____)_____ (_____)_____

Telephone #: (Cellular) (_____)_____ E-mail Address:_____

If Applicable: PINS** Designation: ❑ Yes ❑ No   Court Name/Docket Number:_____

If Applicable: Custody Decree: ❑ Yes ❑ No   Court Name/Docket Number:_____

Do parents/guardians possess child's fingerprints: ❑ Yes ❑ No
   Number of fingers: ❑ 2   ❑ 10 ❑ Other_____

Runaway Child Information

Name: Last _____ First _____ Middle _____

Alias/Nickname: _____   ❑ Male   ❑ Female

Race:_____ DOB: _____ Height: _____ Weight: _____ Hair: _____Eyes:_____

Social Security #: _____ Place of Birth: _____

Physical Characteristics (e.g., glasses, scars, braces, tattoos):_____
_____

School District/Name/Grade: _____
_____

Clothing Description: _____
_____

Describe any noticeable physical or mental abnormalities that the child may have (be specific). _____
_____

Describe any medical problems that the child may have and any medications that he or she must utilize. _____
_____

Describe any drug (including alcohol), mental or any other problems, or dependencies the child may have. _____
_____

---

* Exemplar to be jointly amended by local child welfare and law enforcement agencies for instances in which children run from care.

** Person in Need of Supervision.

(Form continues on next page)

Date/Time/Where Last Seen: _____

_____

If known, describe the motivation for running away (e.g., disagreements with parents, separation or divorce of parents, desire to be independent or alone with a boyfriend/girlfriend).

_____

_____

Has the child ever indicated that he or she would run away? ❑ Yes ❑ No

If yes, provide details. _____

_____

Has the he or she ever run away before?   ❑ Yes ❑ No

If yes, provide details (e.g., when, where, length of time missing, location while missing). _____

_____

_____

Specify all geographical areas that the child has expressed an interest in living. _____

_____

If applicable, describe child's financial resources and methods of payment (e.g., cash, credit cards, checks). Include the names and locations of any financial institutions (e.g., banks, credit card companies) that he or she used prior to running away. Note the type of account used in each institution and account numbers, if known. _____

_____

_____

Do you believe that there is any possibility that any family members, friends, or others are providing aid to the runaway(s)?   ❑ Yes ❑ No

Identify all possibilities by name and location._____

_____

_____

If applicable, specify the type of employment last held by the child and the employer's name and address._____

_____

Describe the child's prior criminal history, if any. Specify arrest charges, locations, and approximate dates._____

_____

Describe any after school activities that the child participated in._____

_____

Describe the child's personality (e.g., friendly, outgoing, withdrawn, shy)._____

_____

_____

Describe the child's general interests (e.g., sports, hobbies, music, reading). _____

_____

_____

Describe the child's career/life goals._____

_____

Describe the child's strengths and weaknesses (e.g., punctual/tardy, enthusiastic/indifferent)._____

_____

_____

(Form continues on next page)

Relationships [to be amended based on child's living arrangements]

Describe the relationship between the child's foster parents (e.g., adversarial/amicable/violent).____

Was there an ongoing or pending custody dispute?   ❏ Yes ❏ No
If yes, provide details. _____

Vehicle Information (if applicable)

Is there a vehicle involved?   ❏ Yes ❏ No
If "Yes," obtain the following descriptive information about vehicle:
Make: _____ Model: _____ Approximate Year: _____ Color: _____
Registration (License Plate) Number: _____ Registration (License Plate) State: _____
Special Identifiers:_____

Investigating Law Enforcement Agency Information

Name of Investigating Law Enforcement Agency:_____

Agency Address:_____

Investigating Officer Name: _____Telephone #: (_____)_____
Describe the last viable leads that were investigated on this case. Include the dates and locations.
_____
_____
_____

Companion Information (if applicable)

If the runaway is believed to be with a companion, provide the following information:
Describe the relationship between the child and companion (e.g., boyfriend, girlfriend, friend, brother, sister, acquaintance)._____

Name: Last _____ First _____Middle: _____

Alias:_____ Maiden Name: _____

Race:_____ Date of Birth: _____ Height: _____ Weight: _____ Hair: _____ Eyes:_____

Social Security #: _____ Place of Birth: _____

Physical Characteristics (e.g., glasses, scars, braces, tattoos):_____

Last Known Address: Street: _____

City/State/ZIP:_____Parent Names: _____

If applicable, cite occupation generally:_____

Specify any noticeable physical or mental abnormalities that the companion may have. Please be specific._____

(Form continues on next page)

Companion's place of birth (municipality, state, and country). _____

_____

Specify all geographical areas that the companion has expressed an interest in living. _____

_____

Describe any drug (including alcohol), mental or any other problems, or dependencies the companion may have. _____

_____

Was there an ongoing or pending custody dispute?   ❑ Yes ❑ No

Do you believe that there is any possibility that any companion family members, friends, or others are providing aid to the runaways?   ❑ Yes ❑ No
Identify all possibilities by name and location. _____

_____

Specify the educational level of the companion (e.g., grade school, high-school graduate, college graduate). If known, include the names and addresses of all schools/colleges attended. _____

_____

Cite any skills, hobbies, or general interests that the companion may have (e.g., computer training, hunting, fishing, sports). _____

_____

Specify the type of employment last held by the companion and the employer's name and address. _____

_____

_____

Describe any deviant or bizarre behavior displayed by the companion (e.g., sexually or physically abusive, violent, paranoid). _____

_____

Describe the companion's self-image (e.g., introvert/extrovert, timid/aggressive, strong/weak). ____

_____

If applicable, describe the type of vehicle that the companion prefers to drive, including the type and manufacturer (e.g., sports car, pickup truck, brand or maker). _____

Describe the companion's prior criminal history, if any. Specify arrest charges, locations, and approximate dates. _____

_____

Describe the companion's career/life goals. _____

_____

Describe the companion's strengths and weaknesses (e.g., punctual/tardy, enthusiastic/indifferent).

_____

_____

If applicable, describe companion's financial resources and methods of payment (e.g., cash, credit cards, checks). Include the names and locations of any financial institutions (e.g., banks, credit card companies) that he or she used prior to the disappearance. Note the type of account used in each institution and account numbers, if known.

_____

_____

Additional Narrative/Background Information _____

_____

New York State Division of Criminal Justice Services Missing and Exploited Children Clearinghouse: Family Abduction Checklist*

Reporting Person Information

Date: _____   ❑ Male   ❑ Female

Name: Last _____ First _____ MI _____

Street Address: _____

City/State/ZIP: _____

Relationship to Child: _____

Telephone #: (Home/Work)
(_____)_____ (_____)_____

Telephone #: (Cellular) (_____)_____ E-mail Address:_____

If Applicable: Custody Decree: ❑ Yes ❑ No   Court Name/Docket Number:_____

Do parents/guardians possess child's fingerprints: ❑ Yes ❑ No
    Number of fingers: ❑ 2   ❑ 10   ❑ Other_____

Missing Child Information

Name: Last _____ First _____ Middle _____

Alias/Nickname: _____   ❑ Male   ❑ Female

Race:_____ DOB: _____ Height: _____ Weight: _____ Hair: _____Eyes:_____

Social Security #: _____ Place of Birth: _____

Physical Characteristics (e.g., glasses, scars, braces, tattoos):_____
_____

School District/Name/Grade: _____
_____

Clothing Description: _____
_____

Describe any noticeable physical or mental abnormalities that the child may have (be specific). _____
_____

Describe any medical problems that the child may have and any medications that he or she must utilize. _____
_____

Describe any after school activities that the child participated in._____
_____

Describe the child's personality (e.g., friendly, outgoing, withdrawn, shy). _____
_____

Describe the child's general interests (e.g., sports, hobbies, music, reading). _____
_____

* Exemplar to be jointly amended by local child welfare and law enforcement agencies for instances in which children are abducted from care.

(Form continues on next page)

Relationships

Describe the relationship between the child and the abductor (e.g., close, distant)._____

_____

Describe the relationship between the child's parents (e.g., adversarial/amicable/violent)._____

_____

If known, describe the motivation for abduction._____

_____

Was there an on-going or pending custody dispute?   ❑ Yes ❑ No
If yes, provide details._____

_____

During any disagreement between the parents, did the abducting parent ever indicate that he or she would use the child(ren) as leverage (e.g., tried to get a child to take sides, threatened to take a child)?   ❑ Yes ❑ No
If yes, provide details._____

_____

Has the abducting parent ever taken the child(ren) before? ❑   Yes   ❑ No
If yes, provide details (e.g., when, where, length of time missing, location while missing)._____

_____

Abductor Information

The abductor is: (Check all that apply)
     ❑ Mother   ❑ Maternal Grandmother   ❑ Other Relative_____
     ❑ Father   ❑ Paternal Grandmother
     ❑ Stepmother   ❑ Maternal Grandfather
     ❑ Stepfather   ❑ Paternal Grandfather

Name: Last _____ First _____ Middle _____

Alias/Nickname: _____ Maiden Name:_____

Race:_____ DOB:_____ Height:_____ Weight:_____ Hair:_____Eyes:_____

Social Security #:_____ Place of Birth:_____

Physical Characteristics (e.g., glasses, scars, braces, tattoos):_____

_____

Occupation (generally):_____

_____

Specify any noticeable physical or mental abnormalities that the abductor may have. Please be specific._____

_____

Cite abductor's place of birth (municipality, state, and country)._____

_____

Specify all geographical areas that the abductor has expressed an interest in living._____

_____

(Form continues on next page)

If the abductor has a regional or foreign accent, please describe._____
_____

Describe any drug (including alcohol), mental or any other problems, or dependencies the abductor may have._____
_____

Is the abductor prone to violence against the: Child(ren) ❑ Yes ❑ No   Parent ❑ Yes ❑ No

Is the abductor from a single-parent home?   ❑ Yes ❑ No

Was the abductor a victim of abuse as a child?   ❑ Yes ❑ No
  If yes, please provide details (e.g., abusers)._____
_____

Do you believe that there any possibility that any family members, friends, or others are providing aid to the abductor (e.g., helping to hide the child[ren])?   ❑ Yes ❑ No
  Identify all possibilities by name and location (continue on the back if necessary)._____
_____

Specify the educational level of the abductor (e.g., grade school, high-school graduate, college graduate). If known, include the names and addresses of all schools/colleges attended._____
_____

Cite any skills, hobbies, or general interests that the abductor may have (e.g., computer training, hunting, fishing, sports)._____
_____

Specify the type of employment last held by the abductor and the employer's name and address.____
_____

Describe any deviant or bizarre behavior displayed by the abductor (e.g., sexually or physically abusive, violent, paranoid)._____
_____

Describe the abductor's self-image (e.g., introvert/extrovert, timid/aggressive, strong/weak).____
_____

Describe the type of vehicle that the abductor prefers to drive, including the type and manufacturer (e.g., sports car, pickup truck, brand or maker)._____
_____

Describe how the abductor generally interacts with the child(ren)._____
_____

Is the abductor religious?   ❑ Yes ❑ No
  If so, provide details (e.g, religious affiliation)._____
_____

Describe the abductor's prior criminal history, if any. Specify arrest charges, locations, and approximate dates._____
_____

Describe the abductor's career/life goals._____
_____

(Form continues on next page)

Describe the abductor's strengths and weaknesses (e.g., punctuality/tardiness, hard worker/lazy, neat/sloppy)._____

Describe the abductors financial resources and methods of payment (e.g., cash, credit cards, checks, loans). Include the names and locations of any financial institutions (e.g., banks, credit card companies) that he or she used prior to the abduction. Note the type of account used in each institution and account numbers, if known._____
_____
_____
_____

Is it believed that there may be other individuals (e.g., new spouse with children from a previous relationship) traveling with the abductor and child(ren)? ❑ Yes ❑ No
  If yes, please identify all by name and provide as much information (e.g., dates of birth, ages, physical descriptions, occupations) as possible._____
_____
_____
_____

Abductor Vehicle Information

Is there a vehicle involved?   ❑ Yes ❑ No
If "Yes," obtain the following descriptive information about vehicle:
Make: _____Model: _____ Approximate Year: _____ Color: _____
Registration (License Plate) Number: _____ Registration (License Plate) State: _____
Special Identifiers:_____

Investigating Law Enforcement Agency Information

Name of Investigating Law Enforcement Agency:_____
_____

Agency Address:_____
_____

Investigating Officer Name: _____Telephone #: (_____)_____
Describe the last viable leads that were investigated on this case. Include the dates and locations.
_____
_____
_____

Additional Narrative/Background Information
_____
_____
_____
_____
_____

State of Illinois Department of Children and Family Services: Missing Child De-Briefing Form*

Procedures 329 Locating and Returning Missing, Runaway, and Abducted Children April 30, 2004—PT 2004.08

Child Name: (Child ID)

Caseworker Name: (Caseworker ID)

Type of Absence:* (ABD   WUK   WCC)   Current (LIVAR)

Dates Missing: From _____ to _____   Date of De-Briefing: _____

Location of De-Briefing: _____

The child's caseworker should ask the child the following questions. Record the child's answers in the space provided. Use the back of the form if necessary.

1) Why did you leave your previous placement?_____

_____

2) Did anyone encourage you to leave?_____

_____

3) Did you tell anyone you were leaving before you left? If so, who did you tell?_____

_____

4) How much money did you have with you when you left?_____

_____

5) What is the first thing you did after you left?_____

_____

6) Where did you go?_____

_____

7) If you were planning to go to a specific place, did you go there?_____

_____

8) With whom did you stay while you were gone?_____

_____

9) How did you survive (i.e., Where did you sleep? Where did your get food? How did you get money?)_____

_____

10) Did you get sick or were you physically hurt or injured while you were gone? ❏Yes   ❏ No
If   so,   describe   your   illness   or   how   and   where   you   were   hurt/injured._____

Did you get medical care anywhere? If so, what care did you get and from where did you get medical care?_____

_____

---

*Available from http://dcfswebresource.prairienet.org/downloads/
pdf.php?d=Procedures_329.

**ABD = abducted; WUK = whereabouts unknown; WCC = whereabouts unknown, periodic contact with caseworker; LIVAR = living arrangements.

(Form continues on next page)

11) Were you sexually active while you were away?   ❑ Yes ❑ No
If so, describe the sexual activity (i.e., when, with whom, what activity, forced or voluntary, etc.).
_____
_____

Did the sexual activity hurt you in any way?_____
_____

For females, do you think you may be pregnant?_____
_____

Note: Any child who reports having engaged in sexual activity must be examined by a doctor within 24 hours of being located. Also, if a child reports being forced to engage in sexual activity, the caseworker must make a report of the assault to the appropriate law enforcement agency.

12) Why (or under what circumstances, e.g., police picked the child up) did you return?_____
_____

13) Have you ever run away before? If so, when and why?_____
_____

14) What was the best thing about being away?_____
_____

15) What the worst thing about being away?_____
_____

16) Do you think you might runaway again in the future? ❑ Yes ❑ No
If so, why would you run away again?_____

What can I (caseworker) or your caregiver do to help you make a decision to not run away in the future?_____
_____

17) Is there anything I can do for you right now to make you feel safe so you won't run away again?
_____
_____

18) If the ward had her/his child with them while missing:
a) How did you meet your child's needs for food, diapers, milk, etc., while you were gone?_____
_____

b) Did your child stay with you all the time you were gone? If not, who cared for your child?_____
_____

c) Who watched your child when you needed a break?_____
_____

d) Did your child need to a see or did the child see a doctor while you were gone?_____
_____

If so, why?_____
_____

e) Does your child need any medical care now?_____
_____

Caseworker's Signature_____Date_____

Supervisor's Approval
Supervisor's Name: _____
Supervisor's Signature:_____
Date of Approval:_____

Children Missing from Care Expert Panel and Reviewers*

The following individuals attended the Child Welfare League of America and the National Center for Missing & Exploited Children Invitational Meeting.

David Barnard
Detective, King County Sheriff's Office CID/Major Crimes Unit, Regional Justice Center, Kent, WA

Roberta Bartik
Commander, Chicago Police Department, Chicago, IL

Patsy Buida
National Foster Care Specialist, Children's Bureau, Washington, DC

Kenneth Buniak
Clearinghouse Manager, New York Division of Criminal Justice Services, Missing and Exploited Children, Albany, NY

Lee Condon
Special Agent Supervisor, Florida Department of Law Enforcement (FDLE) Missing Children Information Clearinghouse, Tallahassee, FL

Mike Cusick
Executive Director, Florida Coalition for Children, Tallahassee, FL

Peggy Daniel
Program Analyst, DHHS—Office of the Inspector General, Office of Evaluation and Inspections, Atlanta, GA

Christine DeVere
Professional Staff, Subcommittee on Human Resources/House Committee on Ways and Means, U.S. House of Representatives, Washington, DC

Judith Dunning
Statewide Coordinator for Missing Children, Illinois Department of Children and Families, Springfield, IL

Celeste Edmunds
Christmas Box House International, Salt Lake City, UT

Nick Gwyn
Longworth House Office Building, Washington, DC

Ruth Huebner
Child Welfare Researcher, Kentucky Cabinet for Families and Children, Office of the Secretary, Frankfort, KY

* Affiliations as of March 2004

S. Kate Johnson
Out-of-Home Care Planner,
Wisconsin Division of Children
and Family Services, Madison, WI

Rick Koca
Founder and CEO, Stand Up for
Kids, San Diego, CA

Michael Lesmann
Field Operations Liaison, Office of
Children's Services, Juneau, AK

Andrea (Ande) Nesmith
Researcher, Chapin Hall Center
for Children, University of
Chicago, Minneapolis, MN

Cathleen Newbanks
Assistant Secretary, Florida
Department of Children and
Families, Tallahassee, FL

Robin Nixon
Director, National Foster Care
Coalition, Connect for Kids,
Washington, DC

Gale Holmes Norman
Child Locator Unit Coordinator,
State of Michigan Family
Independence Agency, Lansing, MI

Rose Perry
Programs Field Representative,
Department of Human Services—
Children and Family Services
Division, Tulsa, OK

James Payne
Judge, Marion Superior Court,
Juvenile Division, Indianapolis, IN

Lee Reed
Officer, Abilene, TX

Jerry Regier
Secretary, Florida Department of
Children and Families,
Tallahassee, FL

Raine Ritchey
Children's Deputy, Board of
Supervisors County of Los
Angeles, Los Angeles, CA s

Thomas Smith
Lieutenant, Collier County
Sheriff's Office/Planning and
Research Unit, Naples, FL

Elizabeth Yore
General Counsel, Illinois
Department of Children and
Family Services, DCFS Legal,
Chicago, IL

CWLA Staff

Kathy Barbell
Senior Program Director, Program
Operations, Washington, DC

Shay Bilchik
President/CEO, Washington, DC

Pamela Day
Director, Standards,
Washington, DC

Alicia Drais Parillo
Washington, DC

Carrie Friedman
Director, NDAS, Washington, DC

Kiyonda Hill
Program Assistant, Washington,
DC

Caren Kaplan
Director, Child and Family
Protection, Washington, DC

Noel Kinder
Program Manager, NDAS,
Washington, DC

Carrie Martin
Program Manager, Standards,
Washington, DC

Linda Morgan
Director, Office of Program
Development and Integration,
Washington, DC

John Sciamanna
Senior Policy Associate,
Washington, DC

John Tuell
Deputy Director, National Center
for Program Leadership,
Washington, DC

Millicent Williams
Director, Foster Care,
Washington, DC

NCMEC Staff

Terri Delaney
Director of Publications,
Alexandria, VA

Marsha Gilmer-Tullis
Director, Family Advocacy
Division, Alexandria, VA

Nancy Hammer
Policy Counsel/Director,
International Division,
Alexandria, VA

Rae Robinson
Family Services Liaison, Family
Advocacy Division, Alexandria, VA

Glossary

Agency—Public or private child-serving entity or other organization providing child welfare or family-centered services, including community-based organizations providing family resources, supports, and education services.

Age-Out—The termination of legal foster care status due to the attainment of adult status at age 18 or older. Publicly funded child welfare services end because a young person has reached the statutory age limit.

Best Practices—Recommended services, supports, interventions, policies, or procedures based on current validated research or expert consensus.

Caregiver—Any individual who provides direct services to children and youth. Caregivers may work independently, as in the case of foster homes or family child care homes, or they may be employees of agencies, including group and residential facilities.

Confidentiality—The protection of information obtained during a services intervention from release to organizations or individuals not entitled to it by law or policy.

Family—Defined broadly, the term includes a variety of family formations, including single-parent and blended families. Family may include birth- or adoptive parents, grandparents, siblings, foster parents, legal guardians, or any other person in a parental role.

Family Foster Care—Essential child welfare service for children and their parents who must live apart from each other for a temporary period of time because of physical abuse, sexual abuse, neglect, emotional maltreatment, or special circumstances. Children are placed in the homes of licensed, trained caregivers.

Independent Living—The development of programs, policies, and services that best support the positive development of youth as adults, citizens, community members, employees, and family members.

Investigation—An inquiry or search by law enforcement and child welfare agencies to determine the location of a child missing from care.

Kinship Care—The full-time nurturing and protection of children by relatives, members of their tribes or clans, godparents, stepparents, or other adults who have a kinship bond with the child.

Kinship Foster Care—The daily parenting care of children by kin as a result of a determination by the court and the public child protective services agency that a child must be separated from his or her parents because of abuse, neglect, dependency, abandonment, or special medical circumstances. In formal kinship care, the court places the child in the legal custody of the child welfare agency, and kin provide full-time care, protection, and nurturing.

Law Enforcement Agency—The agency responsible for investigation of a child who is missing from care at the local, state, or federal level.

Missing-from-Care Episode—Period of time during which a child is missing from out-of-home care as a result of running away, abduction, or being lost in care.

Multidisciplinary Team—A group established among agencies or individuals to promote collaboration and shared decisionmaking regarding the prevention of, response to, investigation of, and recovery of children missing from care.

Out-of-Home Care—Array of services, including family foster care, kinship care, and residential group care, for children who have been placed in the custody of the state and who require living arrangements away from their birthparents.

Partnership—A process of individuals and organizations in a community working together toward a common purpose. All parties have a contribution to and a stake in the outcome.

Permanency Planning—Process through which agencies make planned, systematic efforts to ensure that children are in safe, nurturing family relationships expected to last a lifetime.

Policies—Written requirements that direct the business and service delivery practices of an agency. Policies should carry the approval of the agency's governing or advisory board.

Prevention—The proactive avoidance of missing-from-care episodes.

Procedures—Written guidelines developed by an agency's administration to ensure that operational practices are consistent with board-approved policies.

Protocols—Interagency agreements that delineate joint roles and responsibilities by establishing criteria and procedures for working together on cases in which children are missing from out-of-home care.

Resolution—Completion of the missing-from-care episode, including return, safety and risk assessment, service and permanency planning, and prevention of future episodes.

Respite Care—Temporary relief provided to primary caregivers to reduce stress, support family stability, prevent abuse and neglect, and minimize the need for out-of-home placement.

Return—Retrieval of the child into the physical custody of the child welfare agency.

Safety and Risk Assessment—An assessment of the likelihood that a child is in imminent or future danger of going missing from out-of-home care or will incur harm during a missing-from-care episode. A child is safe if an analysis of all available information leads to the conclusion that the child in his or her living arrangement is not in immediate danger of harm and no interventions are necessary to ensure the child's safety.

Service Plan—An agreement, usually written, developed between the child, the family, the child welfare worker, and other service providers. It outlines the tasks necessary by all individuals to achieve the goals and objectives to sufficiently reduce the risk of future child abuse and neglect, resolve issues that may lead to (or have led to) a missing-from-care episode, and prevent future episodes.

Teaching Interview—A learning tool that is intended to help model the desired competencies while instilling confidence and increasing and reinforcing the knowledge and skills of the recipient.

Workload—The amount of work required to successfully manage a case and bring it to resolution. It is based on the responsibilities assigned to complete a specific task or set of tasks for which the social worker is responsible.

References and Additional Resources

Biehal, N., & Wade, J. (1999). Taking a chance? The risks associated with going missing from substitute care. *Child Abuse Review, 8,* 366–376.

Calhoun, G., Kaplan, C., & Williams, M. (2003). *CWLA best practice guidelines: Child maltreatment in foster care.* Washington, DC: CWLA Press.

Child Welfare League of Amrica. (1995). *Standards of excellence for family foster care services.* Washington, DC: Author.

Child Welfare League of America. (1999a). *Standards of excellence for kinship care services.* Washington, DC: Author.

Child Welfare League of America. (1999b). *Standards of excellence for services for abused and neglected children and their families.* Washington, DC: Author.

Child Welfare League of America. (2004a). *Proceedings of expert panel meeting.* Washington, DC: Author.

Child Welfare League of America. (2004b). *CWLA standards of excellence for residential services.* Washington, DC: Author.

Child Welfare League of America. (2005). *CWLA standards of excellence for transition, independent living, and self-sufficiency services.* Washington, DC: Author.

Courtney, M. E., & Wong, Y. I. (1996). Comparing the timing of exits from substitute care. *Children and Youth Services Review, 18,* 307–334.

Department of Health. (2002). *Children missing from care and from home.* London, UK: Author.

Fasulo, S. J., Cross, T. P., Mosely, P., & Leavey, J. (2002). Adolescent runaway behavior in specialized foster care. *Children and Youth Services Review, 24,* 623–640.

Florida Department of Law Enforcement and Florida Department of Children and Families. (2002). *Operation SafeKids: Results, findings, & recommendations.* Available from http://www.fdle.state.fl.us/publications/safekids_final.pdf.

Finkelhor, D., Hammer, H., & Sedlak, A. J. (2002, October). *National Incidence Studies of Missing, Abducted, Runaway, and Thrownaway Children (NISMART). Nonfamily abducted children: National estimates and characteristices.* Washington, DC: Office of Juvenile Justice and Delinquency Prevention.

Friedman, R. (2002, Winter). The importance of helping the helper. *Best Practice, Next Practice: Family-Centered Child Welfare*, 16–20. Available from http://www.cwresource.org/publications.htm.

Hammer, H., Finkelhor, D., & Sedlak, A. (2002). *Children abducted by family members: National estimates and characteristics*. Washington, DC: U.S. Department of Justice. Available from http://www.ncjrs.org/html/ojjdp/nismart/02/index.html.

Hoff, P. M. (2002). *Family abduction: Prevention and response*. Alexandria, VA: National Center for Missing & Exploited Children.

International Critical Incident Stress Foundation. (n.d.). *Signs and symptoms of critical incident stress*. Available from http://www.icisf.org/CIS.html.

Kaplan, C. (2004). *Children missing from care: An issue brief*. Washington, DC: CWLA Press. Available from http://www.cwla.org/programs/fostercare/childmiss.htm.

Mitchell, J. T. (1983). When disaster strikes...The critical incident stress debriefing. *Journal of Emergency Medical Services, 13*(11), 49–52.

National Center for Missing & Exploited Children. (2000). *Missing and abducted children: A law-enforcement guide to case investigation and program management*. Alexandria, VA: Author.

Ross, T. (2001). *A system in transition: An analysis of New York City's foster care system at the year 2000*. New York: Vera Institute of Justice. Available from http://www.vera.org/publication_pdf/153_223.pdf.

Sedlak, A. J., Finkelhor, D., Hammer, H., & Schultz, D. J. (2002). *National estimates of missing children: An overview*. Washington, DC: U.S. Department of Justice. Available from http://www.ncjrs.org/html/ojjdp/nismart/01/index.html.

Social Exclusion Unit. (2002). *Young runaways*. London: Author. Available from http://www.socialexclusionunit.gov.uk/published.htm.

Turman, K. M. (Ed.). (1995). *Recovery and reunification of missing children: A team approach*. Alexandria, VA: National Center for Missing & Exploited Children.

U.S. Department of Health and Human Services. (2000). Title IV–E Foster Care eligibility reviews and child and family services state plan reviews: Final rule. *Federal Register, 65*(16), 4019–4093.

U.S. Department of Health and Human Services. (n.d.). *Results of the 2001 & 2002 Child and Family Service Reviews*. Available from http://www.acf.hhs.gov/programs/cb/cwrp/results.htm.

Wade, J., & Biehal, N. (1998). *Going missing: Young people absent from care*. Chichester, UK: John Wiley and Sons.

Additional Resources

American Public Human Services Association. (2002). *Missing children: Being prepared when the media call*. Washington, DC: Author. Available from: http://www.aphsa.org/Policy/ChildWelfare.asp.

Bass, D. (1992). *Helping vulnerable youths: Runaway & homeless adolescents in the United States*. Washington, DC: NASW Press.

Biehal, N., & Wade, J. (2002). *Children who go missing: Research, policy and practice*. London: Department of Health. Available from http://www.dfes.gov.uk/qualityprotects/pdfs/missing-children.pdf.

Coco, E. L., & Courtney, J. (1998). A family systems approach for preventing adolescent runaway behavior. *Adolescence, 33*(130), 485–496

Crespi, T. D., & Sabatelli, R. M. (1993). Adolescent runaways and family strife: A conflict-induced differentiation framework. *Adolescence, 28*(112), 867–878.

Finkelhor, D., Hammer, H., & Sedlak, A. J. (2002). *Nonfamily abducted children: National estimates and characteristics*. Washington, DC: U.S. Department of Justice. Available from http://www.ncjrs.org/html/ojjdp/nismart/03/index.html.

Finkelstein, M., Wamsley, M., Currie, D., & Miranda, D. (2004). *Youth who chronically AWOL from foster care: Why they run, where they go, and what can be done*. New York: Vera Institute of Justice. Available from http://www.vera.org/publications/publications_5.asp?publication_id=244.

Hoff, P. M. (1997). *Parental kidnapping: Prevention and remedies*. Washington, DC: American Bar Association. Available from: http://www.abanet.org/ftp/pub/child/pkprevnt.txt.

National Center for Missing & Exploited Children. (1999). *Guidelines for programs to reduce child victimization*. Alexandria, VA: Author.

Office of Juvenile Justice and Delinquency Prevention. (2004). *When your child is missing: A family survival guide*. Washington, DC: Author. Available from http://ojjdp.ncjrs.org/enews/04juvjust/040519.html.

Regehr, C., Leslie, B., Howe, P., & Chau, S. (2000). *Stressors in child welfare practice*. Toronto, Canada: University of Toronto. Available from http://www.cecw-cepb.ca/Pubs/PubsAll.shtml.

Takas, M., & Bass, D. (1996). *Using agency records to find missing children: A guide for law enforcement*. Washington, DC: Office of Juvenile Justice and Delinquency Prevention. Available from http://virlib.ncjrs.org/juv.asp?category=47&subcategory=75.

U.S. Department of Health and Human Services. (2003). *National survey of child and adolescent well-being: Baseline report for one-year-in-foster-care sample*. Washington, DC: Administration on Children, Youth and Families. Available from http://www.acf.hhs.gov/programs/core/ongoing_research/afc/wellbeing_reports.html#wave.

U.S. Department of Health and Human Services. (2003). *Preliminary estimates for FY 2001 as of March 2003. Adoption and Foster Care Analysis and Reporting System (AFCARS)*. Washington, DC: Administration on Children, Youth and Families. Available from http://www.acf.hhs.gov/programs/cb/publications/afcars/report8.htm.

Wade, J. (2003). *Leaving care* (Quality Protects Research Briefing No. 7). London, UK: Department of Health. Available from: http://www.rip.org.uk/publications/researchbriefings.htm.

About the Author and Contributing CWLA Staff Authors

The Author

Susan Dougherty, is Consultant, Dougherty Consultants, Springfield, PA.

Contributing CWLA Staff Authors

Caren Kaplan, ACSW, is Director of Child and Family Protection, Child Welfare League of America, Washington, DC.

Milicent Williams, ACSW, is Director of Foster Care, Child Welfare League of America, Washington, DC.